The
One

W. L. Lloyd-Jones (Buster to his countless friends)
was, until illness incapacitated him a few years
ago, known to thousands as an immensely skilful
and popular vet. Here he tells the story of his life,
in a book that is delightful, funny, moving,
enthralling from cover to cover.

It makes fascinating reading, whether Buster is
feeding lion cubs from a baby's bottle or trying to
persuade Sir Winston Churchill not to stuff his
poodle full of chocolates.

For those who love animals, for those who are
interested in a remarkable life story, this book is
a must.

Available in Fontana by the same author

Come Into My World

The Animals Came in One by One

An autobiography by
Buster Lloyd-Jones

Der liebe Gott hat einen grossen tiergarten
The good God has one large zoo
OLD GERMAN PROVERB

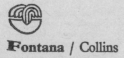

Fontana / Collins

TO DOROTHY AND HAL
who have helped me to live again

First published in England 1966 by
Martin Secker & Warburg Ltd.
First issued in Fontana Books 1968
Seventh Impression May 1974

Copyright © 1966 by W. L. Lloyd-Jones

Made and printed in Great Britain by
William Collins Sons & Co Ltd Glasgow

CONDITIONS OF SALE: This book is sold subject to the
condition that it shall not, by way of trade or
otherwise, be lent, re-sold, hired out or otherwise
circulated without the publisher's prior consent in any
form of binding or cover other than that in which it is
published and without a similar condition including
this condition being imposed on the subsequent
purchaser

ONE

I lay in bed in my small, white room, my bedclothes rumpled, my fists clenched and tears streaming down my face.

It was very late, I knew. The sound of grown-ups who never slept came dimly up the stairs and I had long since heard my sisters say their goodnights and go to their rooms. It must have been at least nine o'clock, the middle of the night, but I was far too upset to sleep. I was four years old and was thinking about the bats.

"Poor things," I was thinking. "They'll be getting caught again. They'll be getting all tangled up. Poor little things!"

It was all the fault of the tennis court. The tennis court was in the garden and was the pride of my father's life. It was a very handsome court with its own umpire's chair in which my father would sit while my sisters played, keeping the score and offering a little gentle encouragement.

"Use your backhand, Lulu," he would shout. "Love Fifteen. Hopeless. Are you blind? Can't you see the ball? Run for it, Betty. Hit it. Fifteen all. Terrible!"

My sisters didn't look forward much to tennis.

All round the court was a wall of fine netting to keep the tennis balls in and this netting was proving a mortal enemy to the bats.

Now bats are highly sensitive to obstacles in their paths and can find their way round a darkened room crisscrossed with wires without touching one. But, for some reason our tennis court netting utterly bamboozled them.

Night after night they would blunder into it and night after night they'd get stuck. We'd find them hanging there in the morning like old socks, their claws hopelessly entangled. Once freed they'd flicker away smartly enough. They didn't seem much the worse for wear.

But that night those bats seemed to me to be the most pathetic of creatures. I cried and cried and at last cried myself to sleep.

Next morning I woke as early as usual, the bats still in my

mind. I got up, slipped out of the house in my pyjamas, and rushed to the tennis court.

There, sure enough, was a bat, well wedged in and just out of reach. I stood on tiptoe, I jumped—still he was too high. So I found an old wooden box, dragged it to the spot, stood on it, and taking the bat's body in one hand, unwound the net from its claws with the other. He was free. Free of the net that is. I still held on tightly.

Bursting with pride and excitement I ran as hard as I could go back to the house, across the hall, up the stairs and into my youngest sister's room. "Look what I've got, look what I've got," I cried. My sister opened her eyes, screamed and pulled the bedclothes over her head. Her voice, muffled and tearful, emerged from the depths of her bed. "You're horrible," she said. "Go away."

My mother was in the room now. "Take him back to the garden," she said. "That's where he belongs."

"But he'll get caught in the net again," I said.

"*Into the garden*," said my mother.

Slowly, reluctantly, I went outside again, held out my hand and opened it. The bat gathered its wits together and, after a moment, was away into the air, swooping, changing course and getting higher and higher.

I was on the verge of tears again and my mother looked at me, amused. "God's zoo!" she said and went back to the house again to get ready, no doubt, for one of her endless committees.

God's Zoo, a very curious, endlessly fascinating place, could have held few more emotional young animals than myself as a small boy.

My parents must have thought they had got themselves a most peculiar child. I thought about nothing but animals. I talked about nothing but animals. I refused to eat pink sugar mice on the highest moral grounds. "Well," I said to Florence, our housemaid, "would you like a sugar mouse to eat *you*?" I thought I had rather a point there.

If ever there was a dispute between a man and an animal I was right there on the animal's side, ready to defend it with my life. There was, for instance, the sad case of Daddy

Isaacson. He was an odd old man with a face fringed with fuzzy ginger whiskers and he wore a tweed trilby hat with the brim turned down and an old clay pipe in the hatband. His trousers were ancient corduroy and tied with string below the knees and he always wore gaiters. He looked like a cartoonist's view of Farmer Giles but his job was, in fact, to creep in at night and empty the cesspools.

One hot afternoon, after a long visit to the local, he lay on a wooden bench on the village green and went to sleep. He was spotted by a male swan whose wife was sitting on her eggs on the island in the pond. The swan advanced, feathers spread and hissing loudly, hauled him off the seat and broke his arm. The shock killed him.

Local feeling ran high against the swan but I was entirely on his side. He was, I said, just scared by Daddy Isaacson. Quite properly. I was rather scared of Daddy Isaacson myself.

My earliest memories are of the animals in and around my parents' house. I remember, for instance, our one-eyed donkey and Jacko, my mongrel, and the newts I collected from the ditches, much more clearly than the adults around the place.

I ached to be of use to the animals. How could I help them? I asked myself. How could I *serve* them? Tears welled into my eyes as I thought of their plight. Where animals were concerned I was a very emotional small boy.

On wet nights I suffered agonies, thinking of all the cats that must be out in the rain. " Poor little things," I would think. " They'll be getting wet through. They'll be catching their *deaths*." And, as soon as no one seemed to be looking, I'd borrow my father's huge black umbrella, creep out of the house and scamper up and down the lane, grabbing any cat I could find. The cats would be furious. They would wriggle and scratch and yowl, but I knew what was best for them and would dump them triumphantly in the empty gardener's cottage that stood in our grounds.

Some nights I had several cats secretly locked up there, yowling to get back to their interrupted love life or their own comfortable firesides and next morning, when I would arrive with milk stolen from the kitchen, they would streak through the open door, across the garden and away. This was always a bitter disappointment. Cats, I thought, were sometimes most ungrateful creatures. But the next rainy night my heart would melt and off I'd go once more.

I remember that when I was four we had chicken for lunch. Suddenly I felt revolted by the thought of eating one of those agreeable and friendly birds I had been feeding only that morning. I flatly refused to eat a bite. " Don't be ridiculous," said my mother. " You'll be eating lamb to-morrow and that was running about too only a short time ago." That did it. I refused to eat the lamb as well. My parents coaxed me and scolded me and sent me straight to my room, but I wasn't eating any nice little lamb or nice little bull or nice little anything else. Nice little vegetables were all right. Luckily enough I didn't mind about them for some reason.

I was a bit young, I suppose, to take such a stand, but actually I have never eaten meat of any kind from that day to this.

As a small boy I could always make friends at once with any animal. I understood them far better than I understood the strange adults in the house. When I was five I was found in a kennel with a ferocious bull mastiff. We had only had him for a short time and the adults, who thought he was vicious, were horrified. I thought they were silly. They didn't *understand* him, that's all.

Throughout my childhood—and for the rest of my life —I had a series of dogs which I loved. The earliest I remember clearly was Paddy, an Irish terrier stray which developed a form of St. Vitus Dance and jerked and quivered the whole time, poor little chap. I loved him the more for it. Once he followed me into chapel and was discovered shaking beside me in the pew. We were both ordered out by Mr. Drinkwater, the sidesman, and I remember the horror of that walk down the aisle, all scandalised eyes upon us, and Paddy shivering and twitching at my heels.

One night there was a thunderstorm. Paddy looked a nervous dog and indeed was. As the thunder crashed over the house, he rushed out and raced across the fields, frightened out of his wits.

He never came back. I always thought the gypsies had got him, but I never quite dared brave their encampment to see. But ever since, whenever I hear thunder, I think of Paddy.

I didn't cry when Paddy ran away. I simply couldn't believe he had gone for good and went about expecting to see him scampering towards me at any moment.

Partly to take my mind off things, one of the gardeners told me about carrier pigeons. They never got lost, he said. Wherever they were, however far away they were, they could always find their way back home. No point in the gypsies stealing one of *them,* he said.

The thought of birds flying free but always coming home again at night, perhaps from the most distant parts of the country, entranced me. So I started buying pigeons with my pocket money.

I had, of course, absurdly romanticised the powers and the characters of carrier pigeons. What's more I had no idea there was more than one variety of pigeon. To me pigeons were just pigeons and I had a blissful time cleaning out a loft that the gardener built for me and sitting watching them busily being pigeons. They bred and soon I was the proud owner of quite a flock.

At last the time came for me to put them to the test and I persuaded my friend, the gardener, to drive me and several boxes and baskets to a common some miles away. I don't think he knew much about pigeons either. I opened the baskets. It was a beautiful picture, the white birds circling against the blue sky, and, thrilling with pride we hurried home, praying we would get there first.

We certainly got there first all right. We waited and waited. No pigeons. We never saw any of them again.

Only one thing made up for the devastating sense of loss. It was getting dark and I had just begun to take in the awful fact that my pigeons had gone for ever, when a young magpie flew in, quite exhausted. I made him comfortable with food and drink and, sadly, went to bed.

Early next morning I hurried back to the loft, hoping against hope. Alas, no pigeons, only a very satisfied magpie who had breakfasted well on pigeon eggs. So the gardener rigged up a cage in the house and this was his home for years. We called him Maggott and he became a great family pet, a voluble talker, a wicked mimic—he was one of the early satirists—and a terrible thief. Maggott came to hate the sight of a packet of soap powder. I had an obsession about cleanliness and the poor magpie endured countless baths.

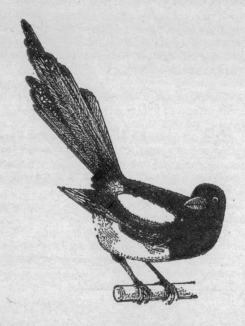

A gawky, happy-go-lucky cross-breed called Jack was soon in Paddy's place at my heels and we'd spend most of our days together, inventing games, chasing each other round the trees, rolling together on the grass.

Then, one awful day, when I was five, Jack jumped over some iron railings, didn't quite make it, and came down hard on one of the spikes. He hung there, impaled and I rushed screaming back to the house for help. One of the gardeners raced over and lifted poor Jack off the spike and together we got him as quickly as we could to the local vet.

I was told to wait outside in the yard while the vet did what had to be done. For a few minutes I did as I was told. Then I couldn't bear it any longer. Quietly, unnoticed by the vet or the gardener, I slipped into the surgery and watched.

The vet was an elderly man, very experienced, very capable. He cleaned the wound thoroughly and then stitched it. He was just finishing when he noticed he had an audience.

"Good heavens, boy," he said. "This is no place for you."

But it *was* the place for me. I had been utterly absorbed, fascinated by every stage of the operation and the old man seemed, to me, wonderful beyond words. From that moment he became my idol.

He was a kindly, understanding man and whenever we brought Jack back for treatment, he let me watch and play around in his surgery.

As for Jack, he was soon happily romping around again and I proudly showed his wound to anyone who would look.

At the same time I took the opportunity of announcing my future plans. When I grew up, I said, I was going to be a vet.

"Ah, well," said my father who had very different plans for his only son, "there's plenty of time to change your mind . . ."

There was plenty of time. He was right about that. But nothing he could have said or done could have changed my mind for a moment.

He tried though. He certainly tried.

TWO

My father couldn't really complain that I was stubborn and strong willed. I got that from him.

He was a stocky dynamic man who loved entertaining and was at his best with crowds about him. He was extremely generous and open handed, quick to help anyone in need and a sucker for a hard-luck story. He could be marvellous company and always had many friends.

But with his family he was strict and rather awesome. He held big, strong views on everything and never compromised, and a man who won't bend a little isn't easy to live with.

There was, for instance, the small matter of the naming of his third child. After two girls had been born he decided that the third was to be a boy. He knew just what he'd call him too. His name would be John.

The third child was duly born and turned out to be yet another girl. My father was extremely displeased and had her christened Palmer after a friend of the family. But in a little while he started calling the little girl John anyway—and everyone else followed suit. So my youngest sister has been called John by her family, her friends and her husband ever since.

Then there was the graver question of his faith. He was a devoutly religious man. He conducted family prayers round the breakfast table every morning and there was a lengthy grace before each meal. He was Chapel and regarded drink as a servant of the devil. There was never any alcohol in our house. On Sundays we went twice to chapel and twice to Sunday school, there was a communal hymn singing for family and servants in the evening and the visiting minister usually came to lunch.

It was this that caused my father's loss of faith. Ministers visited our chapel in rotation and because my father could be excellent company, they often chose to eat with us after the morning service.

On the fatal Sunday it was the turn of Mr. Bloomfield. He was a great friend of my father and was always a welcome guest.

The service began in the usual way with my father booming out the hymns and giving us sharp glances to see that we were really praying and not pretending. Then Mr. Bloomfield mounted the pulpit and began his sermon.

His text, he said, was from Exodus, Chapter 20, verses 8 to 11. "Remember the Sabbath day, to keep it holy. Six days shalt thou labour and do all thy work; But the seventh day is the Sabbath of the Lord thy God; in it thou shalt not do any work, thou, nor thy son, nor thy daughter, thy manservant nor thy maidservant, nor thy cattle, nor thy stranger that is within thy gates . . ."

But there were those in his congregation that day, Mr. Bloomfield went on, who ignored the words of the Lord. There were those who turned the Sabbath into a day of gross over-indulgence, who worked and who made their servants work to produce lavish meals, who drove their motor-cars about the countryside, who used the Sabbath not as a day of rest but a day for gaiety and enjoyment . . .

My father was quiet and thoughtful as we walked home. We always had to walk to church and Sunday school because my father, too, thought it a devilish act to use a car on Sundays and only used his to take the minister from our parish to the next. This car was an enormous beige Sunbeam with brass acetylene lamps and an enormous hood. It must have been colossal, this car, because during the general strike my father got ten people in it at a time perfectly comfortably, to take them to London and back.

When we got back home that day my father excused himself for a moment while he had a word with the cook, then he and Mr. Bloomfield had their usual chat in his study and we assembled in the dining room.

Mr. Bloomfield said grace and the servants brought in the serving plates under their big silver covers. They placed the roast and the vegetables before my father and, we all noticed with some surprise, they placed a separate dish before Mr. Bloomfield. The maid removed the cover with rather a flourish and Mr. Bloomfield blinked down upon two small cold sausages. He looked up in bewilderment at my father who was carving with some relish. "I listened to your sermon," said my father. "We all listened to it. It was very good and I agree with it. With every word. Now then, you practise what you preached. And never ask to come to this house again."

It was a deeply embarrassing meal. Only my father seemed to enjoy his food. The rest of us could hardly bear to look at poor Mr. Bloomfield, pale and thin lipped, manfully eating his cold sausages while the rest of us faced our usual substantial Sunday lunch.

The meal ended at last and my father had another shock for Mr. Bloomfield. He always drove the minister to his next engagement, but not today.

"You'd better set off in good time," said my father. "This is the Sabbath so I cannot take my car out. It's quite a walk to Hounslow . . ."

The minister left on foot. He never returned to our house. And from that day to the end of his life my father never again set foot inside a church. There were no more prayer meetings, no more hymn-singing. He even stopped saying grace before meals. With my father it was all or nothing.

He had been born in a little village in North Wales and had left college at the end of his first year, arriving in London penniless and determined to make his fortune.

He set about it in the classic way, got a job in a dress business in the city and worked his way up. Eventually he took the firm over. He then set about expanding it and ended up a rich man with three large factories.

So my three older sisters and I lived in some style. My parents kept moving—they moved three times before I left home and once more afterwards, each time to remarkably similar houses and all in the same neighbourhood. I suppose this succession of houses must have been a mark of my father's material progress, but looking back they all merge into one big double-fronted house with stables and outhouses and two or three acres of ground. One had a tennis court and one a sunken Italian garden and one a great oak tree with a platform in the branches where I could hide for hours. That was my favourite house. But which was which? What I do know is that I would hardly recognise any of them if I went back. One is a convent now and another is divided into flats and whole roads of modern semis, complete with shops and in one case a pub and in another a telephone exchange, have been built in their gardens.

We were well looked after. We had three gardeners and a cook and a maid and a Japanese nurse for the children and I was called Master Llewellyn, Llewellyn being my Christian name, and was dressed up in white sailor suits complete with cap, lanyards and whistle on summer Sundays and Eton suits with deadly hard white collars on winter Sundays.

I adored the fragile Japanese girl who nursed us. Her name was, of all things, Agnes, which certainly didn't suit her, so we called her by her surname which was Eto—pronounced Ee-to.' Her father worked at a neighbouring big house. We didn't see much of him.

It was Eto who first taught me that herbs weren't just weeds, to be rooted up, but natural medicines with remarkable powers. I remember she was particularly fond of verbena, that wild plant that smells of lemon. Later I was to use it to keep flies and other insects at bay and to repel dogs when bitches were on heat. The idea of drinking the stuff is alarming. But drink it, in large quantities, we did!

We were all very upset when she left to marry the man of her parents' choice. The marriage had been arranged when she was a child and we thought this very hard lines. She didn't, though, and went off happily enough. And years later she returned to show us her five little Japanese boys. I remember thinking they were girls as they all had fringes.

My mother was a handsome, graceful woman who was, in some ways, as determined as my father. She was utterly unsentimental and never mothered us in the accepted sense. No one was going to spoil *her* children. There were times when we would have given a great deal to be spoiled.

She had been one of thirteen children herself and had been brought up in a happy, bustling household in the Cotswolds where her father farmed and ran a livery stable.

All her life she had a passion for animals. I got that from her.

She was a great figure in the life of what she called the village. She was a great one for Good Works as, indeed, was my father. They divided up the local Good Works equally between them, my father taking the Chapel (before Mr. Bloomfield's fatal sermon), the Boy Scouts and the Red Cross, and my mother, Orphans, Dr. Barnardo's Homes, Sick Visiting and Overseas Missions.

She was unyieldingly good living and was deeply shocked when one of us once, in a moment of stress, said s'trewth. "We'll have no foul language in this house," she said.

She herself had only one expression, to be used only in the

15

most dire emergencies. This was "Godfrey Daniel!" spoken in ringing tones.

She had none of the housewifely virtues. She was hopeless at housework, hated cooking and wouldn't do it, and left the drudgery of bringing up her children to others.

Of course she thought she was good at all these things and from time to time insisted on proving it. Such attempts were always disastrous.

When I was born, for instance, she decided that she and she alone should look after me. I was a few weeks old when she pushed me in my pram to the village, did some shopping, sent a telegram, came home, had lunch, then went upstairs to get ready for her afternoon committee. "Where's the baby?" said one of the maids.

"Godfrey Daniel!" said my mother. "I must have left him outside the Post Office."

She rushed, frantic with worry, back to the village. There I was, still outside the Post Office, fast asleep in my pram.

But when it came to her charities she was a model of efficiency and resource—particularly resource.

Every Christmas she would send us out with lanterns to sing carols and collect for the Orphans. Alas, we can't have sung very well. Or perhaps we were too easily discouraged. Anyway we collected very little money.

So my mother had one of her ideas. She collected together a great many jars of home-made jam and set out with us. First she'd ring the door bell. Then, when someone opened the door, she would regally present them with a jar of jam. Then she'd nod to us and we'd begin our carol. At the end she would turn a brilliant smile on to the intimidated citizen in the doorway, who would then fork out handsomely. Our collection was high that Christmas but it had cost my mother an awful lot of jam.

"The village," my mother said, counting our take, "has done very well. . . ."

The village would not have been pleased to hear itself so described. Even in those days Feltham, in Middlesex, liked to think of itself as a country town. A *small* country town, perhaps, but none the less important for all that.

It was a pretty little place, set about with orchards and market gardens, with green open countryside down every wooded lane. There was a quiet little high street leading from the station to the green, and swans sailed like galleons on the pond.

I would buy a pennyworth of aniseed balls from Miss Markham's Sweet Shop, gape open-mouthed at Madam Alaska, a refugee from the Russian Revolution, who would stump down the high street in a Cossack hat, high buttoned tunic and boots, and avoid Jack the Butcher's because Jack, they said, *bit off puppy dogs' tails.*

He did too. I once saw him do it. It was a primitive form of docking for which he charged a fee, but as a little boy I thought he did it because he was a Bad Man. I hated dogs to be docked by any method, but I have to admit that Jack's method, though crude and revolting, must have been moderately efficient.

It was a great place for gypsies and a gypsy king and queen lived in a caravan on the outskirts. I knew that if I was naughty the gypsies would carry me off because my mother had told me so, but I was fascinated by them all the same and I loved their annual fair that would transform little Feltham into a place of great excitement, danger and glamour. There was, as a rule, very little excitement, danger or glamour in Feltham.

As good children of the chapel we were strictly warned against going near the Parish Church. If a service was in progress we must look the other way.

As it happened the vicarage drew me irresistibly. The attraction, not felt by any of the vicar's parishioners or even by the unfortunate vicar himself, was the vicar's wife's herd of pedigree goats.

Mrs. Browell, the vicar's wife, was a brusque, mannish lady who was never seen in church.

Her life revolved round these goats, much to the discomfort of her husband. They were, I thought, beautiful animals but they certainly made the vicarage smell. Even I noticed that. It was, without question, the smelliest vicarage in Middlesex.

Though I hated and feared the butcher's shop I loved the

dairy, run by Mr. and Mrs. Mobbs who had their own cows and made their own butter. Mr. Mobbs taught me how to milk cows and Mrs. Mobbs how to operate the butter churn and they would deliver their fresh milk themselves, clip-clopping along the village streets and through the lanes to the bigger houses on a brightly painted milk cart.

Mr. Mobbs wore a celluloid eye patch and, for a treat, would raise it to show me the livid scar that it hid. His eye, he would say, had been shot out by the Germans. The Germans, I thought, had had a cheek to shoot at Mr. Mobbs.

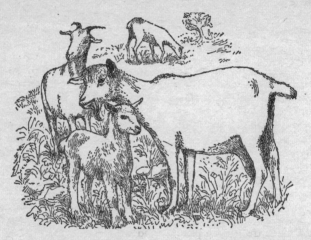

It seems very odd to me now, but my father used to pay the local tradesmen only once a year. I can't imagine why they allowed him to owe them so much for so long, but he was a formidable man, not to be crossed lightly.

It was a useful arrangement for me. Mr. and Mrs. Mobbs sold delicious doughnuts and ice creams and for some months I would take my playmates there and treat them. "My father says please put it on his account," I used to say. I remember my sinking heart the day the Mobbs' bill finally arrived. It was a long bill. Perhaps he wouldn't notice my small contribution. But of course he noticed. "What's this?" he snapped as he carefully checked the list. "And this? And this?" The carpeting that followed left me a sadder and wiser child. It was, indeed, so shattering that I've never liked either cream or cream cakes since.

I remember that little town as being loud with bird song and the countryside around as being alive with small animals of all kinds—rabbits and weasels and hedgehogs and stoats, hares and moles and water rats and foxes, with toads and newts in the ditches and trout in the streams.

You should see Feltham today. Its population has grown from under 10,000 to over 52,000 in my lifetime and most of the old mellow brick houses with their red pantile roofs have been swept away. The high street is twice as wide and one side is dominated by an elaborate new shopping precinct, with stark buildings and modern sculpture for children to clamber over.

Miss Markham's Sweet Shop has long gone. In its place are Woolworths and Boots and Timpsons, supermarkets, banks and a betting shop, Happicraft and Home Charm Stores.

The village pond is still there, neatly concreted now, and nearby is a thriving Bingo hall. Bingo, Bingo, Bingo, shout the posters, Doors open 7.0, Eyes Down, 8.0, Big Cash Prizes. Jack the Butcher and Madam Alaska would have enjoyed that, I feel. My father and Miss Markham would not.

Factories and gravel pits dominate the countryside and concrete and brick are what you notice, not apple blossom and plum trees, open pastures and woods.

It is all a sign of prosperity and indeed Feltham remains a pleasant little town. But for a small boy who lived for animals, the old Feltham was a richer place than the new.

THREE

Neither my father nor my mother could ever believe that anyone was ever ill. They never seemed to be ill themselves and if my sisters or I said we didn't feel well they immediately assumed we were malingering.

"Now then," my father would say briskly. "None of that . . ."

He was a great believer in physical exercise and plenty of fresh air and he saw to it that we got plenty of both. He was particularly keen on my taking full part in all wolf cub activities and was looking forward to seeing me march away to the annual wolf cub camp.

On the morning of the march I felt awful. I said so. My father was exasperated. "Now then," he said. "None of that," and hauled me smartly out of bed.

I felt worse and worse but my pack was strapped on my back and I was hurried off to join the other little boys. The camp was to be at a neighbouring village called Hatton, not very far away, in a field owned by a friend of my father's. It seemed like the end of the world to me that day.

We got there, at last, and then I found we were expected to swim in the river. I obediently undressed, got into my swimming costume, dragged myself to the river bank and jumped in. The water was running quite fast, rushing into a weir a little way downstream and almost at once I was in trouble.

I felt myself being tugged farther and farther towards the terrifying weir and suddenly I was in a whirlpool, swirling round and round and feeling cold hands dragging me under. I screamed. Then strong adult hands were pulling me to safety.

I was dried and put to bed and the cub master anxiously looked at me. "What are all those spots?" he said. No one knew. "Better send for his father," said the cub master.

My father arrived, furious at all the fuss and I was taken home in the deepest disgrace and put to bed. My mother was impatient too, but she sent for a doctor who took one look at me and diagnosed scarlet fever. In the next two weeks the entire troop went down with scarlet fever too. I had generously passed it on to them all.

This was an ordinary enough illness of childhood and I was soon trying to be my father's son again. We could never take anything up like ordinary children. We had to be perfect, to outdo all the other children in the neighbourhood. So we had a coach for tennis, an instructor for riding and another for skating and another for swimming. Normally I would have enjoyed them all—but with my father in the foreground urging us on there was no fun in any of it. Games of any kind became a duty and a drudgery.

Just behind the tennis court was a sunken Italian garden. This had been built by enemy prisoners during the war and very splendid it was with its formal pools and fountains and flower beds.

Most of it was paved and this made it ideal for roller skating. Furthermore, just by turning round in his umpire's chair, my father could supervise the Italian court too and so skating lessons became as great an ordeal as tennis.

" Straighten your shoulders, Betty," my father would shout. " Try to be a bit more graceful, John. *Keep your balance.* Terrible!"

One day I was being taught a step that seemed to be terribly complicated. The instructor was shouting one set of instructions, my father was shouting another. I was skating along, trying to remember what to do with my feet, left over right, right over left, when suddenly I was down with a crash and there was a sharp pain in my leg.

" *Get up, get up,*" bellowed my father. " Don't be such a silly boy. Get *on* with it . . ."

I couldn't get on with it though. I'd broken my leg. My father was furious.

It was set by our elderly family doctor in a little back room under gaslight—set very badly as it turned out. In another six weeks another doctor looked at it and immediately had it re-set, which added six weeks to the time it took to recover. I never did learn that roller skating step and there was to be very little skating or tennis or any other game for me in the years ahead.

One morning, when I was about seven, I woke up with a high temperature and a doctor was called. He gave me some medicine and said I must stay in bed. I rapidly got worse. I found I couldn't move my legs. Then I couldn't move my arms. Then I couldn't sit up or even turn over . . .

The doctor diagnosed sleepy sickness. Then, as the paralysis spread and I slipped into unconsciousness, he made a second diagnosis and this time got it right. I had polio.

Years later I pieced together what happened. My father,

upset no doubt but also disgusted with a boy that was proving so sickly, kept out of the way, but my mother was marvellous. She refused to let me go to hospital, sat up all night with me in the early days and willed me to live. So, largely because of her, I did live.

She wasn't a good nurse in the accepted sense. She was never *tender* and never indulged me in small matters. " If I let you have your own way now," she'd say, "no one will like you when you grow up . . ." and off she'd go to organise another fund-raising effort for the Orphans, leaving me feeling badly done-by.

But if the issue was important she rose magnificently to the occasion. And above all she understood my need for the company of animals. It was because of her that I was allowed to fill my sick room with them.

For weeks, I was critically ill, unconscious a lot of the time. Then, when the immediate danger passed, I was still helpless. Life returned to my limbs, but slowly, slowly, and for a year I did not leave my bed.

Very little was known about polio then, but luckily they did most of the right things. I got electric baths, manipulation, massage and exercises and if some of it didn't do much good it didn't do any harm either.

By a great stroke of luck my mother heard about Sir Herbert Barker and called him in. This was very far-sighted of her because Barker was a hugely controversial figure and anathema to the medical profession.

I remember him as a tall, handsome, greying man with penetrating eyes and strong, intuitive hands that slowly but surely brought my wasted muscles to life again.

He also put my diet right and imposed on me eating habits I kept for the rest of my life. For breakfast, he ordered, I should have fresh orange or lemon juice, brown bread and butter and an apple. That is still my breakfast today. It is the healthiest way to begin a day in spite of the posters that tell you to Go to Work on an Egg. He banished sugar from my life and replaced it with honey.

This inspired my father to keep bees. He was at once tremendously enthusiastic and had six hives installed in the garden. He also bought nets and gloves and read up beekeeping text-books and promptly got very badly stung. The bees also stung for good measure all of my sisters, Batten, the gardener and assorted neighbours.

My father's enthusiasm waned. Bees, he decided, were useful creatures but not worthy of his mettle. After the great stinging outside experts came in whenever necessary to see to the hives. This meant that father's temper was preserved, the bees were happy and that year after year we all had a plentiful supply of home-made honey for our tea.

Barker was a very great man and I used his methods myself in the treatment of paralysed dogs much later. Indeed paralysis in dogs became my special field. I had been paralysed myself. I knew how they felt.

That attack of polio had a profound effect on my life. It shaped my future in an extraordinary way.

As soon as the seriousness of my illness was understood my mother had my bed moved into the drawing room on the ground floor. My father can't have been very pleased about that.

A room on the ground floor had obvious advantages for my mother, who certainly didn't want to be running up and down stairs, but it also had one outstanding advantage for me. The room had a pair of french windows which opened directly on to the garden. These, in spite of protests from everyone who said how *cold* it was, I kept open all the year round. I thought it was cold too but I pretended I liked the cold. The truth was that I wouldn't have kept the animals and birds out of that room for anything in the world.

The room was always full of animals. There were my dogs which slept on my bed. There were the cats, two of which bore litters of kittens on the same night, one in a hat box, the other in a shoe box, and I was appalled when my mother whisked the kittens away. They were all going to Good Homes, she said. I didn't believe her.

There were tortoises, tame rabbits and lizards in a glass case. There was Maggott, the magpie, who strutted and flapped round my bed, talking the whole time, and there were the visitors—the ducks and the bantams who would come and go, the starlings with a heavenly greeny-reddy purple bloom on them, who would sit in a row on the bottom of the bed waiting to be fed. Thrushes would come in too and robins, pugnacious and always ready for a fight. The trees were full of squirrels and I would pretend I had a passion for nuts so that my mother would bring me some every day. They all went to the squirrels and in time they too were coaxed indoors to be fed.

One day Paddy, my twitching Irish terrier, lolloped in with a mole in his mouth. I got it from him and he was a fine, handsome fellow. Before I could get to know him, though, my mother had banished him to the garden again. On another occasion Paddy shepherded in an outraged hedgehog, pushing him forward with his nose right to my bedside. I was delighted with my new visitor. He turned out to be covered in fleas and I was busy removing them when my mother came in. "Godfrey Daniel!" she gasped and out he went too.

When I was not busy coaxing wild animals in I lay for hours watching the wild life of the garden and, as the seasons slowly passed, I gradually began to make sense of what I saw and to understand how nature takes care of its own.

There were the pigeons in the elderberry trees when the fruit was ripe, their breasts stained with the purple juices. It wasn't just that they *liked* elderberries. They were, in fact, storing iron for the winter.

Then there were our cats. Why on earth were they eating that couch grass again? They must know it always made them sick. But of course—that was the whole point. They had a stomach ache and *needed* to be sick.

And here came Paddy, leaping on to the bed and stinking of garlic. How *could* he gorge himself on that wild garlic that grew all over the garden and was cursed by the gardeners? Well, he could because he had to. He had worms and the wild garlic was the certain cure. Now there he was rooting among the wild parsley, chewing it with the air of a small boy taking cod liver oil. He knew that the wild parsley would help to put his kidneys in order. Now I knew it too.

I could hardly realise it then, lying paralysed, but my real education had begun. Later I was to have a governess of my own and later still a succession of teachers. But my best and most valuable teachers were the birds in the trees, the wild

24

life in the undergrowth and my own pets in the garden. I am still learning from them.

They have an instinctive wisdom, a deeply ingrained understanding of nature which men once had too. We have lost it and so, curiously enough, have many dearly loved domestic pets. You will never meet a fat tiger. But you do meet poodles, dachshunds, even alsatians grown fat, flabby and ill through years of over-indulgence. Theirs is too valuable an inheritance to throw away and so, over the years, I have tried to salvage what I could. As a result I have been able to cure animals of all kinds of the diseases of civilisation. It was other animals who taught me how.

At last I was able to go out in a spinal carriage. Actually to leave the house, to go out into the air to feel the sun on my face—it was one of the greatest days of my life.

You rarely see spinal carriages nowadays. They are narrow beds on wheels and you lie flat on your back and look at the sky while someone pushes you along.

This meant that I could now be taken to the Children's Hospital in Great Ormond Street for electrical baths. Three times a week my mother pushed me to the station and got me on the train to London. The journey must have been an ordeal for her and was certainly an ordeal for me. I hated it and longed to be left alone in my sunny bedroom with the dogs and cats and birds and the excitements of the garden.

The specialists in London told my parents that nothing would be better for me than sea water. So they took a flat at Cliftonville and moved there for a whole year.

I loved living by the sea and the sea water certainly did me all the good in the world. The water itself is a great strengthener of muscle and swimming is unmatchable exercise, and later I was to send many limping dogs into the sea.

At first I was carried to the water's edge and lay there in the shallows while the water lapped over me. In time I was able to drag myself farther in and soon I was swimming again and swimming strongly. I could swim long before I could walk again.

Meanwhile my sisters' job was to wheel me around and they were, at any rate at first, very keen. In fact their enthusiasm nearly killed me.

They had pushed me along to Margate for a day and they chose the top of a bank to have a fight over whose turn it was to push. The spinal carriage, untended for a moment, began to roll down the hill and in a split second had gathered speed and was away. It bounced and rattled down that hill, me in it petrified and the screaming girls in frantic pursuit.

At the bottom of the hill was a busy road full of traffic. I went shooting across it at a terrifying speed, missing the traffic in both directions, mounted the far pavement, hit the promenade wall with a crash and turned over. I was flung out in a heap on the promenade. My sisters, shocked and gasping for breath, raced up and bundled me back. I seemed, on taking stock, to be in better shape than them. Either way, one thing we all agreed on. Father must never know . . .

My father was even more impatient with me in a spinal carriage than he had been when I was running round. He could never understand why I didn't like the things he liked. Oysters, for instance.

He loved oysters and would drive to Whitstable to buy really choice ones for the family. I thought they looked like dog's eyes and refused to touch them.

"Don't be so absurd," he would say. "Just try one. Come on, now. Open your mouth and pop one in."

The very idea made me feel sick.

One day he lost patience altogether. "Come on, now," he said. "You'll love them if you'll just *try* one." And, with that, he picked an oyster up and pushed it into my mouth . . .

Horrified I spat it out and it slithered up and down the rubber cover of the spinal carriage, looking more like a dog's eye than ever.

"You *stupid* boy," snapped my father. "You've wasted a *beautiful* oyster . . ." and he ignored me for days.

But as I progressed from a spinal carriage to a bath chair which one could steer oneself and was much more fun, and was clearly getting stronger every day, he got interested again.

My left leg was much stronger than my right, so he had a single-pedal bicycle made so I could get around. He had parallel bars installed in the billiard room so that I could do

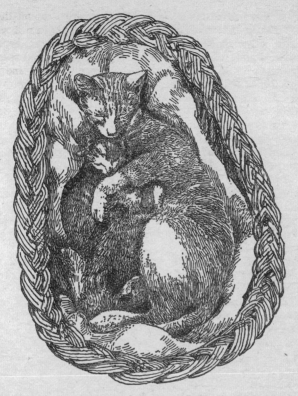

my exercises. He supervised these himself. I had to be the best exerciser that ever was, he'd see to that!

And now, too, I had to catch up on all the schooling I'd lost. I still wasn't able to go away to school, so I had to have a governess.

I didn't look forward to her arrival much. I had read about governesses in books and knew them to be flinty faced, severe ladies, created for the mortification of small boys.

My governess duly arrived and she was no anticlimax. Flinty her face seemed to be. Severe, in spite of her initial smiles, she undoubtedly would prove. I stoically awaited mortification.

But she wasn't all that bad. She came from Scotland and she must have been about 35, though I thought her very old.

She was a forceful lady who wore flat shoes, woollen stockings and tweed skirts and did her hair in dozens and dozens of little rolls like chipolata sausages. When she got angry these used to bounce about all over her head and her voice would get more and more shrill and her Scots more and more broad till I couldn't understand a word she said. She would rap my knuckles with a ruler and make dire threats, but all the same I was fond of her and she, I think, of me.

Certainly she used to push me in my spinal chair for miles into the country, trailing a retinue of dogs, and, wonderfully, she had a wide knowledge of herbs. Her family had been brought up in the country and herbs were their only medicines. So as we trundled along country lanes she would stop to gather this herb and that—aconite for bringing fever down, black current leaves infused to give peaceful sleep, deadly nightshade and bella donna. I can't imagine *what* we used those for!

She failed utterly to teach me the piano or algebra or Latin. But her natural history lessons were a revelation.

Then the old girl stumped back up to Scotland and later we heard she had married. We were astonished. So, I think, was she.

FOUR

By the time I was eleven I was well enough to get back to school and the company of boys of my own age. The prospect dismayed me. For one thing I'd have to leave the animals all *day*. How, I wanted to know, would they manage without me?

My strong humanitarian pleas were cruelly disregarded, I was dressed up in a grey flannel suit, a blue and white tie and a new cap with a Maltese cross on it, and packed off to Richmond Hill School, the newest of new boys.

At first it seemed as bad as I had feared. I was still limping and a bit frail and the other boys found my limp a bit of a giggle. I greatly preferred animals to them. Animals never took the micky.

To my surprise, though, I soon found I was enjoying school. I made friends, I could cope with the work, my limp disappeared entirely, and though I wasn't allowed to play rugger or cricket I found I was one of the best swimmers in the school and a goodish tennis player. This did my morale the world of good.

By the time I was in the sixth form my father allowed me the use of one of the family cars—a little Morris Oxford with a square nose and dicky. It was considered very dashing. About the same time I acquired my first serious girl friend. She had bobbed hair and secretly smoked cigarettes and was also considered very dashing.

Other boys at school used to agonise about what they would do when they left. I used to be surprised by such a curious lack of decision. I told everyone what my future held for me. I was going to be a vet.

The headmaster, a wonderful man called Professor Whitbread and known to us all as Pick, warmly approved. Not so my father.

He had had his own plans for me from the minute I was born. I was to take over the business he had built up, to win new markets, to build new factories, make more massproduced dresses than ever before.

" No," I said. " I'm going to be a vet."

" You're coming into the dress business," he said.

" Never," I said, " I'm going to be a vet."

So I went into the dress business.

The first job my father found for me was assistant to the managing director of Robinson and Cleaver, one of my father's closest friends.

There I was to learn the retail side of the business, get experience in buying and selling, make useful contacts and lay a firm foundation for a prosperous career.

Happily for me my first boss had his own obsession. This was a new kind of life-saving jacket he had patented and he could think of little else.

My job, as it turned out, was to help him test and demonstrate this jacket. I would put it on, have my hands tied behind my back, climb to the top board of Marshall Street swimming baths and jump into the deep end.

I did this every day again and again and again. The jacket worked all right. I didn't drown once.

I then had to demonstrate it to the Air Ministry, to senior R.A.F. officers, to airline executives, to pilots. The top boards I jumped from seemed to get higher and higher. I got tied up more and more firmly. I thought it was great.

My father hadn't any idea that this was how I was spending my time. He assumed I was being trained in the ways of the business world and was disappointed to find I was so unwilling to chat to him about my working day.

It was an easy, well-paid job which gave me a lot of time off and I led a very pleasant life. I became a snappy dresser in Oxford bags and very light sports jackets, flashy red ties and pork pie hats. I slicked my fair hair down with green solidified brilliantine and spent long afternoons on the river.

It was the time of the foxtrot and the quickstep and the tango and of portable gramophones which blared out *Dancing With Tears in My Eyes* and the *Isle of Capri*. I had my own car—a baby Austin—and always carried my own silver flask of whisky, a harmless affectation which made me feel much the smooth man about town.

I had a very daring Jantzen swimming costume with large holes under each arm. This was the latest thing. Then swimming trunks came in. Topless swimming trunks for men! Disgusting! I bought a pair at once.

I worked hard at enjoying myself. I went about with a crowd of youngsters, all as noisy and frivolous as myself. I had a long succession of girl friends and there was dancing and ice-skating, parties and car treasure hunts and dinner at the Trocadero and Noël Coward in *Present Laughter* and it should have been marvellous.

It wasn't though. I was deeply dissatisfied with my life. I felt that time was slipping away, that I was losing my way. I had to make a stand, to face my father and to tell him that I must start veterinary training *NOW*.

But before I could steel myself sufficiently I caught a

curious form of malaria from the kapok in the life-saving jacket and was being closely questioned by puzzled specialists in tropical medicine. How had I caught such a disease without going to the Far East? My work with the life-saving jacket was supposed to be a secret. I said I hadn't any idea.

Then my father found out. He was furious—with his managing director friend, but most of all with me. As soon as I was well again I said firmly that I was going to be a vet this time.

"You're going back into the dress business," he said.

"I'm going to be a *vet*," I said.

So I went back into the dress business.

My new job was as a trainee in a wholesale gown business. I stuck it for a whole year. I had to make appointments to see buyers, take them out to lunch, entertain them and persuade them to come and see our collection.

I wasn't very good at it. I just couldn't get interested. Sometimes I would get on well with a buyer but usually I found we had nothing in common and our conversation would get more and more strained, the pauses longer and longer and any goodwill he may have felt when we met slowly drained away.

I remember taking some dresses to show to the merchandise buyer of a store in Knightsbridge. He received me in a kindly way, asked to see the dresses and watched gravely while I produced them one by one. Then he took me out for a cup of coffee.

"You're new to this business, aren't you," he said.

"How did you know?" I said.

"Well for one thing," he said, "you held up those dresses upside down . . ."

None of this can have been very good for the business.

My relations with my father were as erratic as ever. He could be tremendous company, gay, generous and amusing. Then some small thing would upset him and he wouldn't speak to me for weeks. I would say good morning and good night to him every day and he would look at me as if I was a stranger.

Then the day would come when he would say suddenly, "Be ready tonight at six with two friends. I have a table booked at the Criterion," and the silence would be over. We would have a hilarious night out, a magnificent dinner, quite a lot to drink and he would always be the last to want to get home.

My friends thought he was wonderful. I thought he was wonderful *sometimes*.

One morning I read an advertisement placed by a well-known animal society. They wanted six men over twenty-one for training in animal husbandry. I knew my days in the dress business were numbered.

I applied. I was called in for an interview. Then for another interview. Then for another. They had been inundated with applications and were taking their time making up their minds.

At last, three months later, I got the letter I'd been waiting for. My application had been successful. I should report to begin my course in four weeks' time.

Elated I gave my notice in at work at once. My boss, another friend of my father's, wasn't at all surprised. He had been expecting it for months.

Then I told my sisters, who were delighted, and my mother, who was also pleased. She had known how much of a square peg I'd been in the round hole of the business world.

"But it's going to be ghastly when you tell your father," she said.

I knew it only too well.

For three weeks I put it off. Then, with only a week of my notice to run, I could put it off no longer.

I came back from work and found him sitting in the garden having a drink before dinner. It had been a very hot day and it was a lovely evening.

I told him that I'd applied for a course with the animal society, that I'd been accepted, that I was to start on Monday.

He went white, as he always did when really angry, and his voice became quiet, biting, clipped.

"I won't allow it," he said.

"It's too late," I said. "I've given in my notice at work. I've signed a contract."

"If you leave your job," my father said, "you will get out of this house and never come back."

It was his last word on the subject. He didn't speak to me for the rest of the week.

On the last day I packed a suitcase, came downstairs and found him standing in the hall. Nervously I said goodbye.

He looked at me indifferently, "Goodbye," he said and turned away.

I picked up my case, said an affectionate goodbye to my mother and sisters and the dogs and the cats, took a last look at the garden I loved so much, climbed into my baby Austin and drove away.

I had crossed my personal Rubicon and, as I roared towards London, I felt a great weight lifting off my shoulders.

My new life, my real life, was about to begin.

FIVE

I had already found digs for myself. The day after my father's ultimatum I had gone to Woodford, where the training centre was, and had had a good scout round.

I wasn't very sure how people set about finding digs for themselves, never having had to do it before. So I had picked a likely looking street of small terraced houses and had started ringing door bells.

The housewives who came to the doors were friendly and helpful. No, they couldn't take me in themselves they said, but try the next house along. I was passed from house to house down the street until suddenly there was Mrs. Bushell smiling at me and saying "Yes, certainly you can stay here. Please come in."

Mrs. Bushell was a widow with a sweet, sad face, and a more gentle or loving soul I couldn't have found. Her house was small and shabby and backed on to a railway line, but it was spotlessly kept. There was one other lodger, a young Portuguese called Roy da Cunha who was learning the hotel business. He had the big bedroom at the back and I had a small one at the front. Mrs. Bushell also had a son, Ernest, who was a builder's labourer but who worked hardest at finding excuses not to go to work. His mother worried about him all the time and made Herculean efforts to get him up in the morning.

For thirty shillings a week Mrs. Bushell provided a cooked breakfast, an excellent high tea and some supper and all our meals at weekends. She also did all our laundry.

As I was only getting £2 a week while the course lasted this didn't leave much over. So, feeling I was making the final break with my old life, I sold my car and bought a bike. This transaction gave me some money to draw on whenever I was completely broke. But by cycling to work, cutting out lunch altogether and not going out in the evenings, I had enough over for cigarettes and an occasional beer.

The course proved to be formidable. Our days began at 7.30 in the morning and we would be hard at it until after 6 every evening.

Our first job each day was to muck out the stables, clean the kennels and the cattery, groom the horses and exercise the dogs at the training centre.

Then came lectures for the rest of the morning, a short break for lunch, then more manual work—scrubbing out the animal infirmary and the post-mortem room, the X-ray room and the operating theatre. Then more lectures all afternoon. We attended operations, we were taught to set broken bones, we cleaned and dressed wounds, we medically shod horses, we pored over X-ray plates, we filled mountains of notebooks with notes and took masses of work home every night.

I'd never worked so hard in my life. The world of the dress trade, the expense account lunches, the buttering up of buyers, the easy hours and the high pay, seemed a world away. I looked back with astonishment that I'd stuck it so long.

One evening I arrived back at Mrs. Bushell's with a dead monkey in a carrier bag. I had to dissect him, remove the skeleton and reassemble it so that it worked perfectly. That's what the anatomy lecturer had told me to do. I wasn't looking forward to it.

"What have you there, Mr. Lloyd-Jones?" said Mrs. Bushell. She was always very formal.

"It's my home work, Mrs. Bushell," I said, opening the carrier bag to let her see.

She gave a sharp intake of breath.

"Oh dear!" she said.

"Could I have a bucket?" I said. "And the loan of the gas stove for a couple of hours?"

"Oh dear, oh dear!" she said.

Removing the skeleton wasn't a very nice job. I hated every minute of it. So did Mrs. Bushell. Every now and then she would peep round the kitchen door and retreat again. My fellow lodger stayed firmly upstairs in his room, playing his mandoline and eating the sickly custard apples that were sent to him in large numbers from home.

But once the skeleton had been removed and I had begun wiring all the bones together again Mrs. Bushell got increasingly interested and she would pop into my room in the evenings eager to see how I was getting on.

"How's it going, Mr. Lloyd-Jones?" she would say. "Oh, isn't it lovely . . ."

And by the time it was finished she had become enthusiastic. "Just look, Mr. da Cunha," she said, dragging him in. "It's all finished and working . . ."

"Disgusting!" said Mr. da Cunha.

"It's nothing of the sort," said Mrs. Bushell affronted. "It's *beautiful*."

I agreed with her. I thought it was a masterpiece and kept it for years.

Poor Mrs. Bushell, she was almost crippled with arthritis which became steadily worse. After a while she had to go into hospital, leaving da Cunha and me to do the housework and get Ernest out of bed in the mornings. It was his job to do the breakfasts. After a week of breakfastless mornings we hit on a solution. We tied a string to his bedclothes and led it out of his room and into mine. When my alarm rang and woke me I gave a mighty tug on the string and

Ernest's bedclothes landed on the floor. This meant that every day began with a flaming row from Ernest, but we did get some breakfast.

When Mrs. Bushell came back from hospital she could barely get around. Her church loaned her a wheel-chair and we would push her out for long walks on Sundays. She could cook from her wheel-chair but she couldn't manage the cleaning, so we willingly took over routine household chores and did them, we thought, rather well.

This course finished at last. I sat the exams and waited nervously for the results. Mrs. Bushell was sure I'd passed but I wasn't nearly so confident. Then they came and I was through. It was a marvellous moment and my fellow students and I had a slap-up celebration dinner in a local pub that night.

I was now a qualified lethalist and was entitled to start work to earn a salary again and to wear brown overalls. I hated the title, the overalls and the job I was now qualified to do.

This was to put animals painlessly and scientifically to sleep. This is, of course, a very necessary job, but that doesn't make it any more likeable. In the years ahead I had to put to sleep hundreds of dogs and cats, some of them very ill but others perfectly fit and healthy. It was the one part of the life of a vet that I couldn't bear.

But though this was technically all a young lethalist was *qualified* to do, it was only a small part of the job he actually did. Thankfully even lethalists are mainly concerned with keeping sick animals alive. At any rate this one was.

My first appointment was as lethalist to the animal dispensary in Wimbledon. This was run by an Assistant, who was entitled to wear a white overall. I, in my brown overall, was assistant to the Assistant.

It meant I had to leave dear Mrs. Bushell's. The morning I went she presented me with a large fruit cake, some home-made sweets and heaps of motherly advice.

"Now you will eat properly, Mr. Lloyd-Jones," she said, formal to the end. "None of that skipping lunches. And you'll wrap yourself up well. There's a nasty nip in the air these mornings. Promise you'll wrap yourself up well . . ."

"I promise, Mrs. Bushell," I said.

I was lucky with digs again in Wimbledon. I found a room in a big house where there were ten other lodgers and it was very pleasant, but it wasn't a patch on Mrs. Bushell's.

The food there was substantial enough but Mrs. Bushell would never believe it. Every fortnight she sent me a parcel containing some home-made cakes or fruit pie or some biscuits. When at last the parcels stopped I knew there was something badly wrong. There was. Mrs. Bushell's arthritis was now so bad that she had been sent to a home where she could be properly looked after. She died soon afterwards.

There are fashions in dogs as in everything else and the chic dogs of that time were scotties, spaniels and wire-haired terriers. These lived in great numbers in Wimbledon which was then, as now, a well-to-do, fashion-conscious place, and sometimes looking at our patients for the day, it seemed that the only dogs in the world were scotties, spaniels and wire-haired terriers.

I was astonished how many came in with snake bites. The bitten dogs were astonished too. English dogs don't expect to meet snakes and tend to prod them with their noses when they do. The adders on Wimbledon Common took strong exception to this indignity and were quick to retaliate. Their bites can be nasty.

The Assistant at Wimbledon was a young married man who was only too keen to have an evening off and leave me, strictly against the rules, in charge. Naturally I was delighted.

But my first patient completely threw me. He was a handsome chow with badly weeping eyes. "His eyes have been watering for months," said his owner.

I'd never come across such a thing before so I fell back on a maxim learned early by all homoeopathy students: if in doubt, give n.v. N.V. is nux vomica, a mild stimulant which does no harm at all and gives the student time to think and ask advice.

The chow returned when the Assistant was on duty and he, of course, knew an inverted eyelid when he saw one and performed the necessary minor operation. I have done this operation myself many times since—and often on chows. I don't know why chows' eyelids are so troublesome but they are.

It was at Wimbledon that I treated my first wild animal. This was *really* living.

There was a circus on the common and one of the lionesses was refusing to nurse her two cubs.

Every day for eight days I went along with a baby's bottle, morning and afternoon, and fed them. I sat outside the

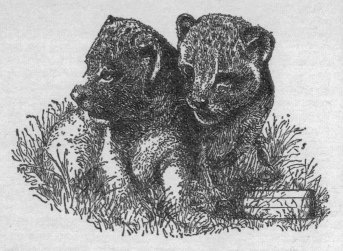

cage. The mother sat, watching warily, inside. The cubs were very greedy and very strong and they struggled and gasped and gurgled as they guzzled the warm milk.

I suppose any of the circus hands could have fed them just as efficiently but I had fallen in love with the cubs and insisted it was a very specialised job that only a real live assistant Assistant could do.

I was very sad the day that the circus left town.

After six months at Wimbledon I was back at the training centre for another crammer course. Again I passed the exams and I was now an Assistant myself, entitled to a white overall and a dispensary of my own. It was a heady moment.

My first dispensary was Stockwell, with Sunday surgeries in the East End once every three weeks—one of them in a street so notorious that the police patrolled in pairs or not at all.

Mosley's black shirts were always at it on Sundays, which was my surgery day, and there would be riots outside the windows as I treated a dog with enteritis or doctored a tom. Luckily enough, though windows all round were broken ours stayed intact.

I was now working in much poorer areas and most of my patients were mongrels and cross-breeds and very fine dogs they were too. Pedigree scotties, spaniels and wire-haired terriers appeared to have become suddenly extinct.

I was appalled by the poverty all round me. Very often the owners were more in need of treatment and of proper feeding than their pets. One day I was called to a house to deliver a goat of her kids. I expected to find her in some kind of out-house, but there she was in the living room of this hovel, calmly watched by two men sitting back smoking pipes.

In the corner, wired off with chicken wire was a sow with a litter. Chickens ran around, quite at home, and small children scampered in and out of the second room where a woman lay, herself in labour. Before I had finished with the goat the woman's child had been born. And this in the heart of London only thirty years ago.

An early patient in the East End was a costermonger's donkey, called, of course, Neddy.

Donkeys are the sweetest natured of all creatures and are naturally strong and resilient, but this one was in a terrible state. His owner had pierced his ears with a red-hot poker to keep away, he said, the evil spirits. The wounds had festered and turned septic.

Quite apart from that the poor beast was in a shocking physical condition, wrongly fed and grossly overworked.

The ears were easy to cure. Persuading the costermonger that he must change the donkey's diet and work him less hard was more difficult.

But in the months that followed he brought Neddy to see me regularly and the change was remarkable. Looking at this sleek, well-fed, affectionate donkey I would sometimes think of my comfortable life in my father's world and know, once again, it was a world well lost.

I had seldom seen my father since leaving home. I'd seen my mother and my sisters, of course, and had sometimes gone to the house when I knew he would be out. They told me he was still bitterly hurt by my defection.

I worried about it from time to time and often wished he could see me, working away in my white jacket, surrounded by animals.

He would surely recognise a happy man when he saw one.

SIX

For five years I worked in animal dispensaries all over London, learning my job as I went along. Dogs and cats were my main patients but any day might also bring rabbits, white mice, goats, a crop-bound hen, a carthorse, a tortoise, a goose, a bush baby, a parrot, a pet monkey or Father Christmas with one of his canaries.

We all called him Father Christmas because of his long white beard. He was a hermit who lived for his canaries. His little house was one large aviary with birds flying from room to room and coming to roost all over the strange, gentle old man.

He would come into the dispensary and give his report. "Jenny is a little better today," he would say, "but little Lucy's rather poorly. Aren't you, Lucy? Not at all yourself today, are you, Lucy?"

"But where is Lucy?" I would say.

"Here," he would reply, reaching into his beard and bringing her out. Little Jenny would be in there too somewhere. So would Dora and Carrie. He always travelled with canaries in his beard.

If I thought he was eccentric what must he have thought of me? He merely carried canaries in his beard. I carried a fruit bat in my pullover.

My fruit bat came from West Africa and his name was Willy. He was brought to the dispensary one day by a merchant seaman. He was a nice little chap, was Willy, like a large furry mouse with an immense spread of wing, but alas, he had hurt one of his eyes.

Blind as a bat is a nonsense phrase. Bats have remarkable eyes and at night see as sharply as owls. Poor Willy, his eye was badly damaged and had to be removed. But he made a good recovery and, as I treated him day after day, he became attached to me. When he was better he clearly didn't want to go home again and after a few days his owner brought him back. " He's *changed*," he said. " He's not happy with me any more."

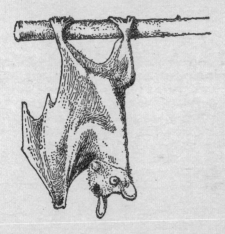

So Willy stayed with me. I became very fond of him. He would swoop about the room in the evening, his great wings flickering, his single eye swivelling to get a wider range of vision, chirruping and squeaking and soaring down to land on my shoulder.

He slept, of course, upside down and he loved to hook on to my mouth. I didn't care so much for this myself. There's not a lot you can do, I found, with a bat in your mouth.

Willy liked company and hated being left at home, so when I went out I'd take him with me. He would snuggle happily inside my pullover and I would forget he was there. One day I was at a party talking to a very attractive girl.

We were getting on well together. Suddenly she pointed at me and screamed. I looked down, surprised, and there was Willy sticking his head out to see what was going on.

"It's only Willy," I said. "He's a fruit bat."

"Oh," she said backing away. "How nice . . ." And she kept as far away as possible for the rest of the evening.

I can never understand why women find bats frightening. They say they are scared they will get tangled in their hair. This is to underestimate bats. They wouldn't dream of entangling themselves in a girl's hair. What's in there that could possibly interest a bat? Willy, certainly, was above such things and I was saddened when, after a while, he died of old age.

Most of my half-days off were spent at the Battersea Dogs' Home. It churned me up to go there and see the appeal in all those sad brown eyes, but I couldn't keep away.

Pedigree dogs are usually all right at Battersea. So are puppies. Either their owners claim them or someone falls in love with them and takes them home.

But middle-aged mongrels—who wants them? The days go by, no one comes to claim them and at last their time is up. They are put down.

Well, the keeper and I became friends and I would persuade him again and again to suspend sentence for another few days while I found a home for one stray after another. Then I would badger everyone I knew to give the poor things a home.

One afternoon there I came across a pen containing an alsatian, a greyhound and two mongrels. "That lot's got to go tomorrow," said the keeper. So I bought the lot myself.

They couldn't get on a bus and I couldn't afford a taxi, so the five of us walked home together. They trotted by my side, delighted to be out and about again.

We hadn't too far to walk because I had recently moved to Chelsea, much to the dismay of my mother. If I lived in Chelsea, she thought, I must be up to no good.

Today Chelsea is highly respectable and very expensive. The art students have been pushed out to Earls Court and beyond and in their place have come debs and young stockbrokers and rising young business executives in need of a

Good Address. The little terrace houses now fetch £15,000 each and E-type Jags, and dashing Alfa Romeos are parked nose to bumper along once humble little side-streets.

But then it was still cheap, colourful, free-and-easy, a marvellous place to be young in and the nearest thing London has ever had to a Left Bank.

I had taken two rooms on the King's Road for £1 a week. They were the top half of a maisonette owned by a glamorous young woman called Elizabeth and no one could have been less like the traditional landlady. What Mrs. Bushell would have made of her I can't think.

Elizabeth knew everyone and everyone knew her. She was warm, amusing, even tempered and delightful company. She had a breathtaking figure, wore clothes beautifully, was always either giving or going to parties. I hadn't met anyone quite like her.

Elizabeth was the most easy-going girl, but even her face fell when she saw me ambling up her stairs with four assorted dogs that day.

"Oh *no*," she said. "Not *four*. Buster, you've gone *too far*."

But she let them stay as I knew she would. Together we put them into a tub and gave them a good wash. We fed them and groomed them and then began to distribute them.

An unwary visitor to the house took one of the mongrels, the second went to the delicatessen shop round the corner and the greyhound went to the greengrocer along the road. Only one was left.

No one would take Rex, the alsatian. So I took him home as a lovely surprise for my mother and father. My mother cautiously took to him—he was a large dog of uncertain temper—and, luckily, he seemed to take to her.

Then he bounded out into the garden where my father was pottering about on the lawn. They looked at each other and it was hate at first sight. Rex growled and leaped, hitting my father on the shoulders and bowling him over. We rushed forward and dragged Rex away but it was not, we felt, a promising beginning.

My mother had her heart set on keeping him and, to my surprise, my father gave in. From that moment he and the dog waged war. My father demanded discipline and obedience. Rex did just as he pleased. My father insisted that Rex should cease instantly from terrorising tradespeople. Rex took his meaning and bit the postman. My father punished him and Rex bit a dinner guest. My father punished him more severely and Rex bit my father.

It was clearly not working out and so at last my mother found another home for him on a farm, where he settled down at once and didn't bite anyone. As he was employed there as a guard dog this was less than satisfactory. No one could ever accuse Rex of being over eager to please.

A few weeks later I came home from the Battersea Dogs' Home with yet another mongrel. He was *almost* a lakeland terrier, almost but not quite, and Elizabeth took one look and fell in love with him.

She already had a pedigree poodle called Silver, a marmalade cat called Giotto and a canary. Now the mongrel, newly named Simon, was adopted too.

Elizabeth was deeply devoted to her pets and, when the war came, evacuated the two dogs to a quiet farm in Bedfordshire.

The poodle couldn't settle, refused his food and pined, so Elizabeth brought him back to London.

Ironically, poor Simon, the mongrel, living in the supposed safety of the countryside, was killed in an air-raid soon afterwards. Giotto was also killed by blast and the canary lost an eye in raids on London, but Silver, the poodle, lived through all the London raids and survived the war unscathed.

The war was getting nearer and the Munich crisis burst on us, completely changing, for the moment, the nature of my work. For years I had been treating pet dogs and cats to make them well. Now, as the crisis worsened, nice friendly people who I knew to be devoted to their pets panicked and brought them in to be destroyed.

I pleaded with them, argued with them, lost my temper but they insisted. Some I managed to find new homes for, but even that was becoming almost impossible. So many had to be put to sleep. On one day alone, when the crisis was at its height I had to destroy fifty dogs and cats. Fifty! It was a black day for me.

But the tension affected us all and back home in Chelsea

the parties multiplied as we set out to enjoy ourselves at all costs. War was coming. We felt we had to make the most of every day of peace left to us.

The Chelsea Arts Ball that year was wilder than ever. The theme was Flaming Youth and we spent days planning our costumes. I went in the end as a French Hussar with tight black trousers and a magnificent white jacket, heavy with gold epaulettes and lashings of gold braiding.

The great hall was packed with tier after tier of youngsters in extravagant fancy dress, dancing and singing and shouting and drinking and making love and then the floats came in, more magnificent than anyone could remember. The final float arrived at midnight. It carried a circle of splendid young men painted gold, supporting a most beautiful young girl, her head thrown back, her arms raised and wearing, it seemed, nothing but her long dark hair. Flaming youth herself.

We cheered and shouted and applauded and suddenly my sister, who was standing next to me, said "Good heavens, it's little Betty Crawford!"

I looked again, and so it was. Betty Crawford who had gone to Sunday school with us in Feltham. Demure and well-behaved Betty, so carefully brought up, who I'd only ever seen in jumpers and tweed skirts and sensible shoes, and there she was in her skin with all of the Albert Hall cheering. We couldn't believe our eyes.

Suddenly everyone was swarming over the floats, tearing them down, and Betty Crawford disappeared into the general mêlée. We fought our way across to her.

"Betty!" we said, not choosing our words as carefully as we might have done. "How lovely to see you!"

Now we were closer she turned out to be wearing rather more than it had first appeared. But it was still hard to know where to look.

"Oh gosh," she said. "You must *swear* not to tell Mummy . . ."

I can't remember much of the rest of that evening except that I completely lost my prized hussar's jacket in the scrum and had to borrow a raincoat to get home in. I got back at 6 a.m. and at 8.30 had to be on duty at the dispensary with a waiting-room full of animals to treat.

The loss of that jacket cost me a great deal. I caught flu which developed into double pneumonia. I was off work for weeks and didn't seem to be getting much better. Then the doctors told me it was essential for me to get to the coast. I needed rest and sea air.

So the Society transferred me to the animal hospital at Brighton.

As soon as I was well enough to travel I left Chelsea and the crowds of friends I had made there and Elizabeth, the most unlikely of landladies and set out for the south coast. With me, a cocker called Gary and a mongrel called Bonzo, both from the Battersea Dogs' Home, and a cat that had walked in one day and stayed.

I took a flat just off the sea front which the animals seemed to like and gradually began to recuperate. And at Brighton, just as in London, my family of pets went on growing. Two other cockers called Penny and Twopence were wished on me by a man who had taken a job in the north. A west highland white called Angus and a black scottie called Robin were brought to me to be put to sleep, which I couldn't bear to do, so they stayed too.

Then a man brought me a sick parakeet with a broken leg. She was a pretty little thing, bright green, yellow and red. I put her leg in a splint and kept her in the flat for a few days to see how she got on.

While she was on the mend some old family friends arrived with their elderly airedale. They were going to Germany for a short holiday, said Hans. Would I look after the dear old dog until they got back.

"But what about the war?" I said.

"Don't be silly," said Hans. "There'll be no war."

Hans was the head of a German travel agency in London. He had lived in England for years and had married an English wife. We all knew how much he loved our country and hated Hitler. We had heard him say so very many times and we were all worried about this rash holiday he was taking.

Then, soon after Hans and his wife arrived in Germany, war was declared. We were never to see either of them again.

But we need not have worried over much. Hans, we learned much later, had been a senior German agent, in charge of recruiting a fifth column organisation. His job had been just a blind. His wife had also been active and they had been recalled to Berlin just in time.

I was left with their affectionate old airedale. I was also left, I soon discovered with the parakeet. Her owner just didn't come back to collect her. My little flat was filling up.

The early days of the war also brought Queenie. Though I couldn't know it at the time, her arrival was to set the pattern of my life for the whole of the war.

When I first saw her she was wedged under the left arm of a tearful middle-aged lady.

She was so *worried* about dear little Queenie, said this lady. What was to become of her now there was a war on? Could I *possibly* look after her for the duration? All right, I said. Well, I must feed her on a special diet, with plenty of cream buns because Queenie loved cream buns, and *do* remember, she said, only to carry her under your *left* arm. Queenie was allergic to right arms.

Now women get pekes wrong too. They are brave, active, and extremely intelligent little dogs, great rabbiters who love to race across open fields and roll in the grass and take on all comers. To be carried everywhere, to be fed on cream buns, to be made a fool of in these ways, what sort of life is that for any dog?

So in her years with me Queenie, promptly rechristened Dinah, was never carried under my right arm. Nor was she carried under my left. She ate a proper diet, lived an active, rumbustious life and had never been more fit or happy.

At the end of the war her owner claimed her again and we said a sorrowful goodbye. A year later, I was walking along the front at Brighton when a plump little peke jumped from under a woman's arm—her left arm!—and, racing across the road, madly clawed at my feet. It was Dinah, reinstated as Queenie. She had recognised me before I had recognised her and, indeed, she was changed. Her silky coat was beautifully groomed and she was plump from a surfeit of cream buns. Her owner hurried across too, scooped her up, talked pleasantly and then we parted once more for the last time. Poor Dinah.

The day after the war was declared I had a completely unexpected visitor. The bell rang, the dogs barked, I opened the door and there stood my father.

I was astonished. We had met briefly from time to time in the past five years when I'd been home to see my mother. But he'd always been cold and distant. Now there he was on my doorstep smiling amicably.

He came in and we talked about this and that in an ordinary civil way. No mention was made of the long breach between us. It was over all the same, thank God, and we both knew it.

Before he left he delivered the message he had set out to bring. It was that I should come home. My mother wanted it and so did he. I said I would like that very much and we parted better friends than we had been for a great many years.

I didn't go at once though. I had come to value my independence, liked having a flat of my own and living my own life.

But civilians in Brighton were no longer welcome. Every week brought a new invasion scare. The front was closed altogether and we could see the fortifications going up and heard about mines being layed offshore and barbed wire and great concrete blocks, for stopping tanks replacing the beach huts and ice-cream kiosks.

Not that we talked about it too much. Careless Talk Costs Lives said the posters and only a few days earlier a mild and gentlemanly clergyman I had often met while exercising my dogs had been marched off to an internment camp. He had been a fifth columnist too.

Then one day in the summer of 1940 everyone in my street was given twenty-four hours to get out.

I had to go home again whether I liked it or not.

SEVEN

It was an odd feeling going back to the house I had left, supposedly for ever, five years before, but my growing family of animals gave me some moral support.

Round my feet, as I rang the doorbell, were six dogs—Penny and Twopence, Angus and Robin, Queenie and the fifth column airedale. I carried two cats in a basket in one hand and the parakeet in a cage in the other.

"There seems," said my father cautiously, "to be rather a lot of you. . . ."

He at once set about organising the deployment of the animals. The cats, the bird and the two smallest dogs, Angus and Robin, could stay in the house, he decided. The four bigger dogs must live in kennels in the stables.

Then, proudly, he showed me how he had prepared the house for the war. Underneath the house were big wine cellars and these had been converted into a comparatively palatial air raid shelter with five bedrooms, a kitchen and a sitting room.

We were to spend most of our nights here in the months ahead. My father, as it turned out, was to spend longer than the rest of us . . .

The next day I set about getting myself into the Army. I knew I wouldn't pass the medical for the fighting services, but I thought the Royal Veterinary Corps would surely take me. Twice I went before medical boards. Both turned me down. The polio of my childhood had left me, they said, hopelessly unfit.

But though they considered me unfit to look after animals in uniform, I was certainly fit enough to look after animals in civilian clothes. So I started looking round for premises to open an animal surgery of my own.

I found a place easily enough—an empty shop at one end of the High Street in Feltham. It was, I thought, ideal. My father, on the other hand, thought the whole plan absurd. The shop was the wrong size, he said, the wrong shape and in the wrong position. But then the whole project was ill-advised. I was, he said, a hopeless businessman. I would lose every penny I put into it and he was certainly not going to throw away any money of *his* on such foolishness. He didn't relish, he said, the prospect of having a bankrupt in the family.

Luckily for me some of our neighbours took a different view of my prospects. A generous and warm-hearted family called Litchfield, three sisters who had always been very kind to me, offered to give me any financial backing I needed, and I was able to go ahead.

I've always enjoyed carpentry, which is just as well as I couldn't afford to hire a professional to do all that had to be done. I moved into the shop with a bag of tools and a load of new wood and put up partitions, built-in cupboards and shelves and finally painted every inch of it white. I now had a waiting room, a surgery and an operating room.

I then filled four big apothecary jars with coloured water, set them in the window, put up my sign—W. L. Lloyd-Jones, Veterinary Practitioner—and opened for business.

That morning I had my first client, a huge bull terrier called George. Now I knew George very well *and* his reputation. He was, in most ways, a charming dog with beautiful manners, quiet, affectionate and lovable. But George lived a double life. Behind that friendly tail-wagging exterior was a notorious cat-killer. When George was around no cat was safe.

But that day he had met his match. He had set about two Siamese cats who had turned round and set about him. As a result poor George's big, white, sheep-like face was lacerated and he was extremely sorry for himself. I cleaned his wounds and dressed them, but some of them were deep and he carried the scars for the rest of his life.

He lived at the far end of the village and every day, as he set out for treatment, the word would fly along the High Street. George was on his way. Every cat owner on his route would dash out, grab the household tom and lock him indoors, and people with cats on their laps in my waiting room would quietly get up and go. I would tell them not to be silly, that George wasn't as bad as all *that*. They never believed me and frankly I didn't really believe it myself.

Wonderfully, my practice was a success right from the start. It grew daily until after a few weeks I could hardly cope with all the work. My father was incredulous. Then, as I got busier and busier, he became interested and then proud of it and started looking in to lend a hand.

He was now in semi-retirement and had a lot of time on his hands, as I soon discovered to my cost. He couldn't keep

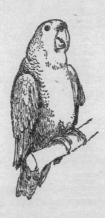

away. He would arrange to meet his friends there, insisted on taking over the books and once again I heard the familiar voice of authority.

"There's nothing wrong with that dog that some regular exercise wouldn't cure," he would boom as I examined a bitch with enteritis. Or "Jaundice? Rubbish, boy. Just needs a good dose of salts . . ."

It was at this time that two of my closest friends came into my life.

Pollyo came first.

My assistant at that time, Valerie Higgins, had been in charge of Pets' Corner in the London Zoo and still had many friends there. One day she told me that one of the Amazon parrots had bitten his keeper and was under sentence of death.

I immediately got in touch with the zoo. Could I have the parrot? Certainly, they said. As soon as you like.

So two days later Valerie arrived with Pollyo in a cage.

He was a magnificent old bird, about sixty-five years old, a vivid green with bright, alert eyes, and we all admired him immensely.

" According to the keeper," said Valerie, " he was given to the zoo by the Prince of Wales."

" She's a vicious one," said her keeper. " She'll get her teeth into you if she can."

From Pollyo came a cackle of derisive laughter and then he began to swear. He swore most foully and with great expression.

" The Prince of Wales?" said my mother faintly. " Indeed!"

One thing the keeper had been very sure about was Pollyo's character. He had impressed on Valerie the need for great caution. On no account were we to let Pollyo out of his cage. He was a very dangerous bird.

That night, when everyone was in bed, I softly played the gramophone, carefully opened the cage and sat on a nearby chair.

Pollyo came to the door, looked around, hopped on to the table, waddled across and flopped down on my knee. I sat perfectly still while he made an inspection of my trousers, my jacket, my tie. Gradually he climbed on to my shoulders and gave my face a thorough inspection. He explored my nostrils and my ears and my mouth. He carefully examined each of my eyelashes, looking into each eye, raising and lowering the lids with his beak. Satisfied, he relaxed and from then onwards became part of the family.

He was particularly fond of Wanda and Wanda of him. This was very proper. Both, after all, were reformed juvenile delinquents. Both had been under sentence of death. They had much in common.

Wanda was a Javanese monkey from a private monkey house a few miles away. The owner was desperately short of food for the monkeys and some had to go.

Now I had always wanted a monkey, so I got myself there as quickly as I could.

Wanda was sitting glowering in her cage. One look at me and she went mad, hissing and grimacing and jumping with rage. I loved her on sight.

" She's a vicious one," said her keeper. " She'll get her teeth into you if she can."

Wanda bared her teeth and scowled and gibbered and her amber eyes flashed fear and hatred. I thought her very beautiful.

We got her into the cage we had brought without being bitten, though Wanda did her best, and I drove her blissfully back home. I was the one who was blissful. She seemed to hate every minute of it.

I kept her cage in the surgery so that I could spend as much time as possible with her. Gradually Wanda and I got to know each other and the great day came when I felt I could let her out. I opened the cage door—and at that moment was called to the phone. I was only gone a few seconds but that was long enough for Wanda.

Immediately she swung herself on to the shelves which were laden with my hard-come-by stock of emulsions, linaments and medicines and seized on them with joy, hurling bottle after bottle against the opposite wall.

By the time I got back, my surgery, always fanatically neat and white, was a shambles, the floor littered with broken glass, the walls dripping with my precious medicines.

She saw me and redoubled her efforts, chattering away with the thrill and excitement of it all.

I was bursting with genuine fury. "WANDA!" I bellowed, slamming my hand on the desk.

She froze with surprise. She had never heard me raise my voice before and her face puckered with astonishment. Then, swiftly, she swung down from the shelf and into my arms making funny little " er-er-er" noises in her throat.

From that moment she was my slave and constant companion. We walked hand in hand to visit the dogs kennelled in the stables and she rode on my shoulder into the village. She loved to watch operations and would peer knowingly into dogs' mouths and ears as she had seen me do. Visitors to my surgery had no difficulty in telling which of us was the vet. I was the one in the white coat.

One day George, the bull terrier, arrived for a final treatment. His wounds had almost healed now and he was full of beans.

Wanda liked dogs and would swing on to their backs, pat them, wrestle with them on the floor. So she was prepared to like George too.

He, however, took her for a cat and, with a growl deep in the back of his throat, jumped at her. She screamed, swung on to a high shelf and shrieked and grimaced at him, making ferocious faces and gestures, *daring* him to come up and get her. He barked and snapped below, infuriated by such uncat-like behaviour.

I got him out of the room, calmed him down and sent him off home, then returned to placate Wanda. But never again did she trust a white dog.

The raids on London had now begun in earnest and Feltham was getting a battering. I was made area officer for something called N.A.R.P.A.C.—National Air Raid Precautions Animal Committee—and as soon as a raid got under way I would be out, with my tin hat on, trying to rescue animals from the wreckage of what had been happy and secure homes . . .

It was a heart-breaking job.

I returned home again and again covered with bites and scratches, bringing with me dogs and cats half crazed with fear and shock.

Some would be badly injured and many had glass splinters deeply embedded in their skin. All were now homeless. Sometimes their owners had been killed. Sometimes they could not be traced. All had two immediate needs—a good meal and somewhere to sleep.

Luckily there were plenty of outhouses at home and I fixed up a cattery and built more and more kennels so that animal refugees could stay until they were claimed or new homes could be found. Some of them came for the night and stayed for years.

Normally my father would have been the first to welcome them, but things weren't well with him. Things weren't well at all . . .

His visits to the surgery had already stopped. This hadn't worried me. He had many other interests to keep him busy.

But gradually he lost interest in other things too. He began to spend more and more of his time in the house and eventually he stopped going out altogether.

Then one night he went to bed as usual in the cellar and next day wouldn't come up again. He stayed down there for six months, getting more disturbed and physically sicker day by day.

At last his doctor insisted that he should be removed to a hospital, where he died a few weeks later. At the time of his death he had not spoken to me for more than a year, though we lived in the same house and saw each other daily.

He had been a strange man, a difficult man, erratic, proud, unforgiving. I had been a grievous disappointment to him.

I wish we had parted friends.

EIGHT

In any civilisation a large population of domestic pets has always been a sign of security, prosperity and peace.

But when the wind blows cold, when belts are tightened and sacrifices must be made, the pets are the first to go.

Between the wars, in spite of the depression, England probably had more pets per head of population than any country in the world. In the south, particularly, there were few households without a pet of some kind.

Almost overnight all that changed. The phoney war was bleak enough for the nation's cats and dogs, but as soon as the nation got down to waging war in earnest their world crumbled completely.

The men went off to war and the women to war work, the children were evacuated and the old settled patterns of family life were, for the moment, abandoned.

With the family gone there was clearly no place for the family pets. So all over the country they were put to sleep in their thousands.

Their owners were often desperately upset by what they were having to do. But there seemed—and indeed there was —no alternative.

Some breeds suffered more than others. Big dogs, for instance, have big appetites and during the war their owners had trouble enough feeding themselves. An alsatian could happily eat an entire family's meat ration for a week in one day. So who could, without enormous trouble, keep an alsatian.

Then there were dachshunds. As soon as the war started the dachshunds began to feature in political cartoons as wicked, cowardly, treacherous, evil German sausage dogs, opposing the gallant British bulldog. No one, you might think, could have taken this kind of routine propaganda literally—but a great many did. In an instant the clever, affectionate little dachshund became the most unpopular dog in the country. People threw things at them in the street, chased them, kicked them. Dachshund owners were looked upon as dangerously unpatriotic.

So they were brought to me every week, healthy, lively little dachshunds, no longer wanted and bewildered by the sudden withdrawal of affection.

They came to me to be destroyed and I couldn't bring myself to do it. I usually found myself bringing them home to join a pack of dogs that had already outgrown the space we had.

Indeed the accommodation problem became so acute that we soon realised that we would have to move. Now that my father was gone the house was too large for my mother, the one sister still at home and myself, and the garden and out-houses were far too small for all the dogs and cats that increased in numbers week by week. So we decided to look for a smaller house with a bigger garden, and an impossible task it seemed to be.

If the house was small enough the garden would be too small and if the garden was big enough the house would turn out to be much too big.

Then we heard about Clymping Dene.

I had known Clymping Dene all my life. It was a very large old house and it had an enormous garden—about ten acres of it. It was a wonderful garden too, totally unlike the formal, landscaped gardens that my father took pleasure in.

He demanded lawns like velvet, strict flower-beds with flowers in military formations, orderly paths and immaculate

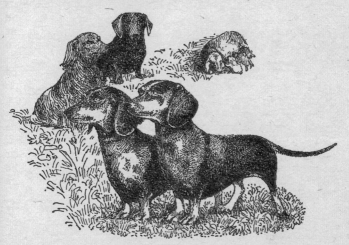

paved courts. In my father's view plants, like children, should do exactly as they were told.

But Clymping Dene was *my* idea of a garden. There was a spinney and a paddock and a colossal kitchen garden and wide stretches of evergreen wilderness. There was a huge lake, twenty-one feet deep, set about with reeds and wild undergrowth, and there were magnificent trees everywhere. It was a beautiful spot, and the lake was treasured by those weekend fishermen lucky enough to have permission to fish there.

There were, what's more, big stables, a lot of outhouses and two empty cottages. It was perfect—but for the size of the house.

Luckily, the house had been divided into four separate

units and, just when our need was greatest, we heard that the first two floors were vacant—and that whoever took the first two floors got the garden. All of it. All ten magnificent acres.

The minute the lease could be drawn up my mother and I moved in. We could hardly believe our luck.

With us, of course, went Wanda and Pollyo and a large number of dogs and cats. There was plenty of room for them already but I was expecting further guests. So the first job was to build as many kennels in the outhouses as possible.

I set about this at once, sawing and hammering away in every minute I could spare from the surgery. Wood was strictly rationed, but clients gave me planks and odd bits of timber and I managed. I put wire partitions into the outhouses and the cottages, built a cattery on the site of an old tennis court.

My mother watched the work progressing with something approaching dismay. "But this is absurd," she said. "You can't possibly need all *that* space . . ." I said that we would, but privately I thought she was right.

She wasn't though. Even before the work was finished the deluge was on us.

The news of empty kennels spread with a speed that astonished and alarmed me. At first in ones and twos, then in dozens, then in hundreds, the pet owners of London and the Home Counties heard that there was after all an alternative to putting their pets to sleep. They would send them to me.

They wrote, they phoned, they travelled miles to see me, begging, pleading, often weeping. Would I please, *please,* take their pets for the duration.

The pack of dogs grew daily until the kennels were bursting at the seams. Before long I had sixty dachshunds alone. Then there were almost a hundred others of all shapes and sizes as well as dozens of cats. And still they came.

It was an extraordinary family of animals that gathered to live out the war in Clymping Dene.

Just as many of their owners had gone from sheltered lives in comfortable suburbs, where privacy was prized and respected, to barrack rooms where privacy was unheard of, so their animals found themselves living a rumbustious new communal life. They lived together, slept together, played together, ate together. And they got on with each other beautifully.

It was a matter of constant wonder to me that from their first day none of the dogs ever pined or fought. They struck up new and sometimes curious friendships. High-born thoroughbreds palled up with rough-and-tumble mongrels; Jack, a tiny Jack Russell terrier, and Fridge, a towering champion greyhound, became inseparable. Dogs and cats that had been fastidious eaters, turning up their noses at unaccustomed foods, tucked in to anything put before them with gusto. Overweight dogs fined down. Neurotic dogs became less highly strung. And they all had a great deal of fun.

For me the day began at 6.30 a.m., making my rounds with Wanda on my shoulder. We saw every animal and if any were sick they would be isolated and treated. Then there was the day's food to be thought of, morning exercise organised and kennel maids to be briefed, and then off for my morning surgery.

When I got home at night there were the evening rounds to be made and the day's crises to be dealt with and then, if there was a raid, it would be out again in my tin hat, looking for bombed-out and injured animals. Sometimes I wouldn't get home again until 6.30 next morning, just in time to make the morning rounds again.

One day a horse arrived and took up residence in the paddock. She was joined by two ponies who came from the nearby gypsies' encampment. The gypsies said the ponies needed a rest and they certainly did. I was happy to let them stay and two months later the gypsies came back and took them away again. The horse, a little chestnut mare who had spent her pre-war days drawing a trap for the children of a rich family, missed them.

Then a distressed woman rang to say that she had just been bombed out and would I take her family pet for just a few weeks until her family got somewhere to live. The pet, she said, would be no trouble, no trouble at all. Bring it down, I said.

She arrived, that afternoon, bringing with her a sheep on a lead. He was called, she said, Benjamin. He was a dear creature, she said. Her children were going to miss him dreadfully. They had brought him up from a lamb and they loved him dearly. The sheep baa-ed sorrowfully and their leavetaking was sad to see.

Well, I hadn't a separate sheep pen so there was only one thing for it. Benjamin would have to go into the stables with the larger dogs. I led him in, petted him a bit, introduced him round to the others and left him.

Next day I opened the doors to let the dogs out for their morning run in the paddock. They rushed out, as they

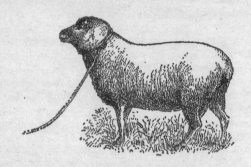

always did, and were followed by Benjamin, trotting as hard as he could, indignant at being left behind.

The dogs rushed round the paddock. Benjamin trotted gamely at their heels. They rolled over in the grass, wrestled, chased their tails. Benjamin stood looking puzzled but willing to learn. Before the week was out he thought he was a dog too and the dogs accepted him as one of themselves— a bit slow, perhaps, a bit dopey poor chap, but all right when you got to know him.

Every weekend his owner's children came to see him, played with him, made a big fuss of him and departed sadly. After a few months the family was together again in a new house and Benjamin went home, wagging his tail and baa-ing all the way down the drive.

Animals continued to arrive. A note would come from the

station saying there was an animal waiting for me and I would hurry over and find a large dog with a small note saying would I please look after Butch until after the war? Or a small basket would be delivered anonymously with a kitten inside.

I vividly remember the day one cat arrived at the station. She wore a great big bow and a message round her neck which read "Please do keep me alive. My name is Rapunzel."

I just hadn't room for her. This one, I decided, *must* be put down. But she was obviously exhausted after her long journey so she was taken to the surgery and fed. I always hated the job, but I'd fixed the day when the deed must be done. To my astonishment, when I opened the lethal bin, there was Rapunzel already. She had made a nice warm bed for herself and was curled up, asleep. I just couldn't bring myself to put her to sleep, and she lived on for another fourteen years.

She used to follow me everywhere—on buses, on trains, and once, to my embarrassment, I found her walking beside me down Piccadilly.

But Rapunzel was certainly a great deal more predictable than Tasha, one of the borzoi bitches.

She was the dumbest of dumb blondes. She would race at a breathtaking speed round and round the paddock, then fly up to you and, where any other dog would have slowed down and stopped, she would go right on, bowling you over and racing on without any reduction in speed. She was a born hit-and-run driver.

Tasha was a compulsive eater and she was also a prodigious jumper and these combined to make constant trouble for me. You would think she was safely shut in but she would gracefully vault a seven-foot gate and be away, scouring every rubbish bin between Clymping Dene and Bedfont. You could follow her progress by going from one overturned bin to the next.

Borzois are Russian greyhounds and have barrel chests and tiny waists. This always gives them a hungry look. Again and again I would get a telephone call from a distant household. "I have a half-starved dog here with your name on its collar," an angry dog-loving English voice would say, and it would be Tasha who, after being well fed at home, had been gorging herself silly on other people's meagre wartime scraps.

When her time came she chose to whelp in the most alarming place. She had a perfectly good, warm, dry, secluded kennel, but she preferred to have her puppies in the lake. Not on the banks, you understand. In the lake itself.

She waded in, lay down and, her long blonde hair floating like Ophelia's, began giving birth.

One of the kennel maids gave the alarm and we rushed to the water's edge in time to rescue the first, then the second, then the third of the puppies. She had produced five before we got her to the bank and then she went on to produce another eight. They were beautiful puppies too—three of them grew up to be champions. But those first five must be the only borzois ever to be born underwater.

I had, as it happened, quite a few champions among my big, noisy family and one of them came to me by a curious route.

Mary Merrall, the actress, had two wire-haired terriers which she adored. I had known them ever since they were puppies and when, one day, they disappeared she rang me up. She was very upset and I said I'd try to find them.

In those days stolen dogs very often turned up on sale at absurd prices in Club Row, the East End street market, so the following Sunday morning I went along.

I'd never been before and I wished I hadn't gone then. I hated seeing all the caged birds and the pathetic-looking mongrels, tentatively wagging their tails and beseeching passers-by to give them a home. Mary's wire-haired terriers were nowhere to be seen, but right at the end of the market was a pathetic little dachshund, spattered with mud and covered with fleas, tethered by a rusty chain. She was being offered for sale by a man who looked as shabby and as ill as she did.

The first anti-dachshund hysteria was over, but they remained the nation's most unpopular breed and I couldn't bear to see her sitting there, so woebegone and no chance of a sale. I asked how much she was. Thirty bob said the man. Done, I said.

Back home I washed her, and treated her for a bad skin

condition and canker, got rid of her fleas, fed her, gave her a name—" Shush " we called her for reasons I can't remember —and, as she got slowly back into condition, I realised that she was a very good-looking bitch.

Not long afterwards a breeder, who had called in for a chat, saw her in the garden. " Good heavens," he said. " Isn't that Champion Tormaid of Loxwood?"

" *Is* it?" I said, astonished.

And so it proved to be.

Now Tormaid of Loxwood was a very distinguished dachshund champion from a very fine kennel. If she had been stolen I would be able to return her. I made inquiries at once—but she hadn't been stolen. She'd been given away . . . And given away . . . And given away.

The owner had dispersed the kennel when the war started and had given two of the best dachshunds to her chauffeur. He had then been called up and had given them away in turn. And this one, the best of the lot, had been passed from hand to hand until at last she had found her way to Club Row.

She was a dear affectionate creature and stayed with me until she died. She found herself in rumbustious, harum-scarum company at Clymping Dene where none of the dogs stood on ceremony or had any respect for a champion's breeding or high social standing.

She was happy, all the same. After her recent experiences in Club Row she knew only too well how the other half lived.

Boozer was another dachshund with no illusions about life elsewhere.

He had been bred in superior kennels and had been sold to a nice, kindly and well-off couple. And from that moment his life was a misery.

His owners weren't cruel. But like many other busy people, living and working in big cities, they should never have owned a dog.

Boozer was shut up in their flat all day, usually alone. Both husband and wife were working and in the evenings they liked to go out. The little dog got very little affection and even less fresh air and exercise. At last even the small amount of time his owners could spare him turned out to be too much and they decided to sell him. One of their neighbours, long scandalised on Boozer's behalf, rang me at once. I agreed to buy him and the neighbour brought him down to Clymping Dene.

He was a sorry sight—thin, miserable, painfully nervous. His nails were so long that he could hardly walk—a sure sign that a dog hasn't had enough exercise. He was terrified of everything, the Good Samaritan neighbour, the kennel maids and, most of all, the other dogs. He'd hardly ever seen another dog. Finding so many around him at once was obviously a nightmare.

Tasha didn't help. I tried to introduce Boozer to the others gradually, but the first time I let him out into the paddock Tasha came flying past, doing her racing car act, knocked him flying and broke his leg. So for the next few weeks the little chap hobbled about in splints.

Gradually, though, he settled down. His coat became glossy, his eyes bright, he completely lost his hangdog look.

In time there wasn't a happier or more gregarious dog in the place. He won prize after prize at dog shows and embarked on a long and fruitful career as a stud dog. In the next few years he was to father at least two hundred puppies . . . I only hope that none of them had the ill luck to go to the kind of nice, kindly, well-off people who had bought Boozer as a pet and treated him as a pretty, woolly toy.

NINE

My greatest problem, of course, was food. Our own rations were small, but for domestic pets there were no rations at all, which was all right for a family with one dog or cat—but I had two hundred of them to get fed every day.

We did our best to make ourselves as self-supporting as possible. I bought six goats to provide milk for sick dogs and once they got into form, there was sometimes enough over for all of the cats and for some of the other dogs. Rich, nutritious milk it was.

The kitchen garden was a godsend, and provided enough potatoes, turnips, carrots, tomatoes, cucumbers, marrows and green vegetables to last a good part of the year and we had a small orchard which produced apples, plums and cherries.

I also gathered together a few chickens which set to and laid eggs staunchly and a bantam or two which loyally did their best though their eggs were far too small to be much help. I also bought a dozen Khaki Campbells for the lake, quite excited at the thought of collecting fresh duck eggs every day too.

Alas, the ducks were infuriatingly unco-operative. Although I had houses built for them they completely ignored them and laid their eggs in the most inaccessible places. They were prolific layers too. Should we by chance see one within reach we would wade in, but the bottom of the lake was a sticky mass of mud and rotted leaves and, though we got many a duckling, we never got a whole egg to shore.

Happily the lake was full of fish and provided us with a steady supply of carp, perch and pike. The cats, of course, were delighted and the dogs got their share as well. After initial reservations they got to like or, at least, tolerate a fish diet. Fish is very good for animals, so I was very grateful to the lake.

All this was a help—but it was far from enough, and getting the rest became a matter of begging and borrowing. We never, to my recollection, actually had to steal.

I was deeply touched to discover how many friends the dogs and cats had made. People for miles around rallied to us. They queued for hours for a few biscuits, a cube or two of Oxo, and for the tiny amount of dog's meat that sometimes went on sale. People made long and tedious journeys to bring us their kitchen scraps. Anything edible, however meagre, was very, very welcome.

So, as the war years went by, we managed. No animal ever went hungry.

The six goats—Dena, Nellie, Katie, Blackie, Snowie and Filtness (who was rather grand and always used her pedigree name)—became very much part of the family. They had the run of the paddock and were on chummy terms with the dogs.

Goats can be very temperamental and sometimes one of them could take offence and blatantly sulk, holding her milk back and ignoring whoever was in disfavour. They never kept it up for long, though, and I got very fond of them.

I was fond, too, of the bantams. Ordinary hens are all right, and I had one, a very fussy lady called Zazu Pits, for years. She was a cross between a Rhode Island Red and a White Sussex, which made her a sort of beige. Miss Pitts was brighter than most hens, but even she wasn't what you would call companionable. Bantams, however, are much better company. They are such handsome little birds and once you get to know them you come to realise just how strong their personalities can be. They make very good pets, but with a bantam stalking about the living-room you can't be too houseproud. Birds are clever creatures. Some can be taught to speak, others to count, others to respond to their names. But none of them can be house trained.

You can't house train a rabbit either, try as you may. But you can get attached to them all the same and the deliberate introduction of myxomatosis, which almost wiped out the European rabbit, was a shameful barbarity.

When, a few years later, I saw them dying in every field, their heads grotesquely swollen, I thought of the pretty, gentle creatures that lodged with us at Clymping Dene, so placid and so unteachable. Only two things ever held their attention for a moment—eating and mating. Still, they are both absorbing occupations. A great many people think of little else either. We can't feel too superior.

The rabbits were pure-bred and beautiful, with lovely long ears and long soft coats. They came from a rabbitry a few miles away, owned by a couple who were moving. They asked me if I would look after the rabbits until they were settled somewhere else. I agreed, built a series of huge hutches on a stretch of grass near the cattery, and along they came.

There were just two dozen of them when they arrived but they bred like—well, like rabbits. A year later, when their owners had established themselves on a farm and took them back, the rabbits had multiplied exceedingly.

Wanda was pleased with the rabbits, visiting them regularly and making faces at them through the wire. But she was far, far more pleased with another new arrival.

A pair of Rhesus monkeys called Jack and Jill lived a few miles away, doted on by the young man who owned them but loathed by his wife. Inevitably he was called up and the minute he was safely on the train his wife hurried to the local

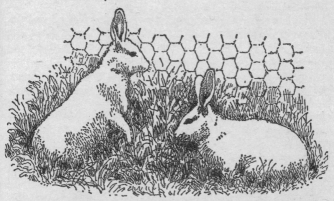

paper to put in an ad. " For Sale ", it read, " Pair of Rhesus monkeys . . . Tame and Affectionate."

Now Rhesus monkeys are handsome fellows with crew cuts and alert, humorous faces. They are highly intelligent and adroit and have been voted the mammal most likely to succeed. So I bought this pair. They would, I thought, be nice company for Wanda.

As it turned out Jack and Jill weren't all that tame or affectionate. Indeed they were a bit sullen. Nevertheless Wanda fell hopelessly in love with Jack. She would scream at him, give him huge cuddles and spend hours grooming him with her fingers—much to the displeasure of Jill.

But both Jill and Jack were thoroughly intimidated by Wanda. She thought she was being infinitely subtle and tried everything she could think of to win Jack over and placate Jill at the same time. One day we saw her hurrying from the orchard, the pouches of her cheeks swollen with cherries. She produced them with a flourish, pressed them on Jill and then, when Jill started cautiously eating them, flung herself on Jack, making the most uninhibited passes I have ever seen. Jill hesitated, glowered, and then went on eating the cherries.

At about the same time a client brought me Bimbo. He knew I liked monkeys, he said, and he was sure I'd love Bimbo. He then left rather hurriedly.

Bimbo was a West African green monkey and he was truly vicious. Given time and quiet privacy he could have been taught to trust and like us, but time and privacy, like everything else at that time, were in short supply and Bimbo remained the worst-tempered animal in the place. I soon understood why my client wanted him out of the house.

Wanda couldn't stand him and neither could Jack or Jill. Neither could any of the other animals. Indeed the only creature who had a good word for him was an extremely pretty kennelmaid called Gloria. She adored him. In return he screeched at her, rattled his cake with rage and tried to tear her hair out. "Pretty little chap," she would say lovingly.

Then a fifth monkey arrived—a Woolly monkey—and the extraordinary thing is that I can't remember a thing about him. I can't remember where he came from or where he went, what he looked like or what he was called. Well, life's like that. Some monkeys you remember, others you don't, but I can't help feeling that this one can't have had a very strong personality.

After about a year Gloria asked if she could take Bimbo home. She thought he wasn't properly appreciated at Clymping Dene. I was delighted to see the little chap go—it was one less mouth to feed. And soon afterwards I found a new home for Jack and Jill, too. Wanda pined for Jack for about half an hour and then forgot him. It had been the love of her life, but you can't grieve over things for *ever*.

Love, indeed, was a problem that was always with us. The dogs and cats were, like rabbits, only too keen on increasing their numbers. We tried to separate bitches and queen cats as they came on heat, but love will find a way and there were some strange matings.

I had one exceptionally valuable pekinese in the kennels, a beautiful haughty little bitch, and on instructions from her doting owner I sent her off to be mated with one of her few social equals, an exclusive pekinese champion of great renown.

She returned after her state visit well pleased with herself and soon proved to be satisfactorily in whelp.

Her pregnancy was normal and uneventful and five enchanting puppies were born. Her owner was thrilled. "They are the most beautiful peke puppies I've ever seen," she said.

But after a few days I began to wonder and after a fortnight, the truth could not be denied. The lordly peke had not been the father at all. The father, plainly, undeniably and lamentably was Boozer.

With a sinking heart I broke the bad news. The lady was very cross, very cross indeed. But the puppies were so pretty she couldn't stay cross for long.

The five of them grew up with long dachshund bodies and squashed little peke faces. They were adorable.

I still see the son of one of these dachsenese scampering along the seafront at Brighton on sunny days. Boozer, I know, would be proud of him.

Always randy and exceptionally fecund, old Boozer did his best at all times to provide still more mouths for us to feed. But it's curious how quickly one forgets the struggle we had to keep going, the air-raids and the long sleepless nights, the whimpering pet dogs in the wreckage of their houses and the half-starved shell-shocked cats living wild on bomb sites, and remembers instead brief interludes of sunshine and happiness.

In 1942, for instance, I organised a Dog Show at Clymping Dene to raise money for the Prisoners of War Fund and the Red Cross. It was a beautiful day and the Germans left us alone and we all forgot the war for a while.

A small R.A.F. band played, the gardens looked delightful, the dogs, the cats, the rabbits and the monkeys were on their best behaviour and only the Khaki Campbells disgraced themselves. The day before we had cut and rolled the lawn until it looked immaculate. But the ducks in their usual unco-operative way had settled on the lawn that night and on the morning of the show you could hardly see the grass for feathers.

They kept well out of the way for the rest of the day, and, by the time we had counted the takings and found we had raised more than three hundred pounds, I had forgiven them. With ladies of the village in their best hats, the dogs parading in the ring, the sideshows and the white elephant stall, the music playing, the sun shining and the gentle sound of tea cups chinking, it could not have been more peaceful. But what places it in my mind so uniquely in the middle of the war was the sad incident of the lemon.

Just before the dog show the lemon came by post. The luxury of it was beyond belief. I had not even seen one since the beginning of the war, when I ate them as most people eat apples.

Wanda was with me when I opened the parcel and she went mad when she saw it. So, feeling it was true love on my part, I cut it in half, giving her one bit and wolfing the other myself.

It was delicious but it was to prove the most expensive fruit I've ever eaten. Next day came a letter from my lemon-sending friend saying that she had forgotten to mention that this was one of three precious lemons that had come into her hands. The other two had been raffled for charity, each one fetching about £10. She did hope mine would do as well at the Dog Show.

Quietly I put £10 in the kitty. Wanda, at any rate, thought it a bargain.

TEN

Not all the dogs and cats survived the war. Some—like the elderly fifth column airedale—died of old age and natural causes. Others were killed by enemy action.

There were weeks when the raids seemed to get longer and more severe every night and nearly always, when the new day dawned, I would get settling another batch of injured or shaken animals into the already packed kennels.

Some weren't easy to collect. One cat, indeed, took me three and a half weeks to coax from the ruins of his home. Every time I got near he shot up the chimney which was still standing. Day after day I would go back to try again and at last I took some chloroform with me, soaked a pad of cotton wool and placed it at the chimney mouth. After a while the poor thing staggered out, half doped.

I caught him, popped him with relief into the basket, took

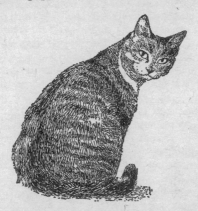

him home and lodged him in the cattery. Only a week later he was sleek, gentle and loving again.

One life gone, eight to go . . .

A few nights later there was an even worse raid than usual and I spent hours digging in the debris of what had been a pleasant street of semi-detached houses, with the howls of buried dogs and cats urging me on. I had put three badly injured dogs to sleep the minute I found them that night and had taken another seven dogs and two cats back to Clymping Dene.

I dressed their wounds and pacified them as best I could, gave them a meal and then lodged them for the night in the gardener's cottage and went back to the house to get some sleep myself.

The raid was still going on and as I lay listening to the planes droning overhead, the ack-ack batteries blasting away, I began to worry about the new arrivals. They must be very frightened out there, I thought, after all they'd been through. So after a while I got up, dressed again, and went out to bring them into the house.

I had just stepped inside the cottage when there was a heart-stopping thud that shook the cottage to its foundations. There was a moment of silence and then a rending, a crash of glass and some isolated cries. I at once thought the house had been hit and rushed to the door. It was jammed.

Now fire bombs were falling and, with the blackout curtains open, I could see the house still, apparently, standing. I could see, too, the eyes of the rescued dogs, peering at me from the far side of the room. They were quiet and trusting. They had more courage than I had the rest of that night.

At 7 a.m. next morning a kennel maid came down to milk the goats and I shouted to her that the door was jammed. She ran for help and I was, at last, released.

Near the goat house was a deep crater and inside the crater was an unexploded oil bomb. The goat house itself and one other outhouse were damaged and four dachshunds, a sweet mongrel called Rags, and Snowie, the goat, had been killed.

As always during raids the other dogs had been quiet, relaxed and apparently unafraid. That morning they were as full of high spirits as ever. I think they gave each other confidence and courage. I only wished they could have given some to me.

The oil bomb lay there, silent and menacing and the police ordered me to evacuate. I could hardly move about two hundred dogs and cats, not to mention a waggonload of monkeys, rabbits and goats, two donkeys and a horse very far. So my mother and sister moved out and stayed with some friends and I moved the cats and goats as far from the crater as possible and all the dogs came into the house.

They slept in every room, on the stairs, in the bathroom, in the lavatory. You couldn't move for dogs.

The electricity was already off. The wires had been damaged in the raid. Now they turned off the water and the gas as well. And that night the rain came down in sheets, and the lake rose and flooded the garden.

I came downstairs next morning clambering over dogs every inch of the way, looked out of the window and saw the Khaki Campbells swimming gaily past and the gardens one sheet of water.

Then the water started coming into the house and all the dogs had to be packed upstairs.

Thankfully I saw from the upstairs window that the water hadn't reached the cats yet. Nor did it. That afternoon it began to subside, next day the bomb disposal unit came, the bomb was emasculated, the electricity, gas and water were reconnected, my mother and sister returned to clean up the house and the dogs went back to their kennels. I slept well that night.

Petrol, of course, was strictly rationed. I had a small allocation mainly for collecting injured animals in air-raids, and there was none over for visiting animals too sick to be brought to me, or distant kennels or farms or piggeries with a sow in litter.

Luckily, I had a staunch ally in the village who could often come to my aid in moments of crisis. This was the village undertaker.

He was a kindly, cheerful man, a great dog-lover, and he had at his disposal a hearse. "If I can ever give you a lift," he said, "just let me know . . ." I took him at his word.

I would let him know where I had to go. He would let me know where he had to go. And time and again we found we could fit both journeys together.

So off we'd go, trundling in mournful dignity through the countryside. Sometimes I would have sick animals to collect. Sometimes I would be taking a recuperating animal home again. Often there would be dogs or cats or even farm animals in the back.

We caused a sensation in some suburban streets. "After you'd gone last week," one jolly housewife told me later, "all the neighbours came in with long faces. I couldn't understand it. They stood round talking in whispers and asking me who'd gone. Then I remembered the hearse. 'Don't be daft,' I said, 'it was only the vet!'"

The problem of getting to and from the surgery in the village was that so many of my animals insisted on coming too.

Wanda couldn't be left behind. Rapunzel wouldn't be left behind. If they came Pollyo had to come. And usually a couple of dogs would join them too.

I had a travelling basket made which could go either in the car or the bus. They would all hurry to get inside it,

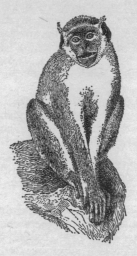

jostling for a good seat and thrilled by the prospect of a journey.

One evening I was half way home with the basket full to the brim with my pets when we were caught by a raid. We had to get off the road so we took refuge in the first pub we came to.

Inside the basket that night were Wanda, Rapunzel, Pollyo and two dachshunds called Baron and Baroness. They seemed quite happy so I put the basket down by the bar and got myself a drink.

There's nothing like going through an air-raid together for making friends and within half an hour I felt I'd known everyone in the bar all my life. Drinks were flowing freely, we laughed and talked and got increasingly merry. Suddenly there was a scream from the corner. The entire bar fell silent for a moment and then there was a roar of laughter.

Wanda, growing bored, had pushed her arms and her feet through the wicker work and was slowly crossing the floor, a grotesque monster with a square wicker body, no head and four hairy legs.

I opened the basket and got her out and she sat on my shoulder, surprised but delighted to find she was such a hit.

Someone offered her a glass of rum which she knocked back in one swallow. I protested but she was given another and another. Then she was cavorting round the room, jumping on people's shoulders, dancing on the bar, stealing every drink she could lay her hands on. The place was in an uproar.

When I at last got her home she could hardly stand. She was given porridge for her supper and slowly, deliberately she turned it upside down on her head. Then with porridge dripping all over her, she hiccupped and went to sleep. She was as drunk as a lord.

I cleaned her up and put her in her basket to sleep it off and then made my evening rounds.

To my dismay Titmus was missing.

Titmus was a large black tom that had been brought in for skin treatment. I'd taken him much against my wishes as we were so overcrowded, but his owner was a very over-powering lady. She gave me one look and I didn't dare refuse.

Now Titmus had chewed his way out of the pen and had disappeared into the night.

I telephoned the owner at once. "*What*!" she roared. "I'll be over at once," and slammed down the phone.

She was there in half an hour, her mild, intimidated husband bringing up the rear, and the minute she saw me she produced a large pair of scissors. I paled and backed away. I could understand her feeling cross but surely not as cross as *that*. She advanced, snipping the scissors loudly in the air. "This will bring him in," she said, snipping away. "He always comes for his food when he hears the scissors."

So the three of us fanned out across the gardens and the

surrounding fields in the pitch darkness, none of us able to show the smallest light. "Tit, tit, tit," called the husband. Snip, snip, snip went his wife. And not a sign of Titmus did we see.

At last we returned to the cattery, the lady furious and still snipping away, the husband silent, me worn out. And there, back in the pen, was Titmus, perfectly content after his evening stroll.

"You naughty puss," said the lady, almost purring with pleasure and relief. I loved Titmus too at that moment. I hadn't trusted those scissors.

In any pack of dogs you are bound to have your favourites and of all the sixty dachshunds, the one I loved most was a lively little black and tan called Alice.

One day another Alice arrived, a plump, matronly little dachshund whose owner had left London for Scotland. After a few weeks this lady wrote to say she was now settled in Glasgow and would I please send Alice. So I asked one of the kennel maids to take Alice to London and put her on the train to Glasgow.

That evening I came back from the surgery and made my evening rounds. My black and tan Alice was nowhere to be seen but there was plump Alice tucking into her dinner with her usual gusto.

The wrong Alice was on the Glasgow train.

Still in my gumboots and overalls I grabbed the other Alice, rushed to the station, and caught the next train to town. I got to Euston just in time, found my Alice sitting looking disgruntled in a basket in the guard's van, swopped the dogs over and caught the underground to Waterloo.

At Charing Cross the train stopped and we were told to get out. A raid had started and no one was allowed to leave the platform.

An hour passed and I began to get claustrophobia. "What a dear little dog," said a well-dressed city gentleman, beaming at Alice. "Can I hold her?" I handed Alice over and she was promptly sick all over his well-cut Crombie. Silently he handed her back again.

Time dragged by. Then the all-clear went and the station doors were opened again. I walked to Chelsea where Ursula

Bloom and her husband Commander Gower-Robinson, friends as well as clients, had a flat. She put me in her spare room and then the sirens went again. The raid was renewed with vigour. One tremendous explosion shattered the bedroom window and Alice and I dived under the bed. We stayed there for what little was left of the night.

When I at last got home I was exhausted, emotionally and physically. Alice, however, was in the highest spirits.

But not for long. Not for very long. Ten days later the dachshunds were playing in the paddock when a random bomb fell nearby.

There wasn't much damage, there wasn't much noise. Alice was the only one killed.

ELEVEN

Clymping Dene had one wartime visitor we could all have done without.

It came unasked and unannounced, stayed two years and made a flaming nuisance of itself most of the time. It was greatly disliked by all the animals, by my tolerant mother and sister, by most visitors to the house, by the local police who I called in to evict it, and by me.

The visitor was a poltergeist.

Now you may not believe in poltergeists and neither, I must say, did I. But let me tell you what happened.

Soon after I had moved into the house I was walking across the garden when a stone flew past my head and landed with a thump on the grass.

I whipped round to see who had thrown it but, apart from Queenie and Rapunzel, there wasn't a soul in sight. I didn't think it could have been them. Then another whizzed by and another. Whoever my assailant was kept himself well hidden.

Still, there were lots of trees about—it was good ambushing country—and I didn't think any more about it.

Next day it happened again. And the day after that. Soon every time I went into the garden I had stones thrown at me. None ever hit me. Whoever it was was a rotten shot.

What began to worry me was the complete absence of anyone who could have been doing any throwing. At one time I thought it might be Wanda, but she was often with me when the stones flew by.

We were too far from our boundaries for the stones to have come from outside the grounds and often too far from the house for the stones to have come from there.

I was beginning to understand what it was to be non-plussed. I was far from plussed too when the organ started up in the night.

I started hearing it in my bedroom at about 3 a.m. Not only did it wake me but it awoke any dogs that were sleeping in my room—and there were usually three or four. Their hackles would rise, they would growl, whine and quiver with fear until I got out of bed, put the light on, opened the door to show them no one was there. Knowing no one was there pacified them but it hardly pacified *me*. It just made things worse.

Then my mother and my sister began to hear the organ and notice the stones. We had an Army padre billeted on us at the time and he said it was all rubbish. So one night we exchanged bedrooms. In the middle of the night he woke me up. "We can change back again now," he said. "I can't get to sleep because of that wretched organ."

After a week or two I called in the police. If a practical joker was at large, I thought, we'd better catch him at it.

They gave me their instructions and hid themselves in the trees. At a given time I had to walk from the house to the stables. I did so—and the stones came down fast and furious.

The police were nonplussed too.

I began to believe that the house really was haunted, though the ghost, if it was a ghost, seemed to be suffering from arrested development. Apart from the organ, which it played rather well, its little tricks were all those beloved of small boys everywhere. It was always, for instance, ringing the bell and running away. And after a while it began to vary the target for its stone throwing and aim for the windows. This time its aim was better. Several were broken.

There was an elderly Irish priest in the village whom I knew well. I'd treated his airedale after she had got mauled a bit in a fight and several times for skin trouble. So I asked his advice.

He didn't bat an eyelid. "I'll be round sometime to-morrow," he said.

He came round next day and went from room to room making the sign of the cross in holy water in each, then settled down for a chat about his airedale. She was, I was pleased to hear, much better now. And so, I was even more pleased to discover, was the house. For three days there were no stones, no organ recitals, no bells ringing.

Then, tentatively at first but with slowly increasing confidence, the whole thing started up again.

Thump went the stones on the grass, crash went another broken window, and that very angry sound was me losing my temper.

As time went by, though, I got more or less used to it. Once I realised that I wasn't going to be actually hit. I didn't mind so much about the stones and anyway I had too much on my mind to worry about small boys, ghosts or no ghosts.

But one day a visitor who had been rather shaken by a near miss suggested I call in an association of spiritualists. I was given a telephone number to ring and I rang it. And so I had more visitors, two very matter-of-fact, down-to-earth women, who looked round the house, listened to the story and said, yes, I had poltergeists. They weren't in the slightest way dramatic about it. They might easily have been telling me I had mice.

They took possession of my bedroom for an hour or so and when they left they took my poltergeist with them. Anyway, there wasn't another peep out of it from that moment.

It was a relief, I can tell you. Not long afterwards I heard Professor Joad talking about poltergeists on the Brains Trust. One of them, he said, had thrown a bit of coal at him and given him a black eye. So it could have been worse. I might have got a poltergeist with a better aim . . .

TWELVE

Many, many times I wanted to say, right, that's enough, I can take no more animals for the moment. But my animal family went on growing all the same.

I didn't at all mind the tortoises arriving. They are self-sufficient creatures and can forage for their own food. First two came, then a third and a fourth and in the end I had

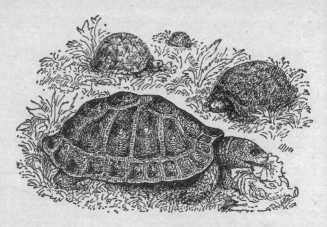

seven roaming round the gardens, taking a quiet, mannerly interest in our affairs. They were no trouble.

But my heart did sink a bit when I discovered that a client of mine, who had just died, had left me her entire aviary of more than a hundred budgerigars.

They were pretty things, pale blue and white and green and yellow—but bird seed was hard to get too. I could have coped with three or four. But a hundred! Rarely can a generously meant bequest have been received so glumly.

However I built an aviary round a small tree near the house. Three of the walls and the room were wood painted white, the fourth wall was wire. The tree stuck out of the top but its lower branches were inside and were at once laden down with budgerigars.

I just couldn't feed them all so I gave them away as fast as I could. They countered by breeding as fast as *they* could. It was like running on the spot. But I won. Almost everyone I knew ended up with one of those budgies. Finally I was left with a dozen or so and with those I was happy.

Three parrots arrived to stay a while too. They had to live inside the house—parrots need a warm room. They got on

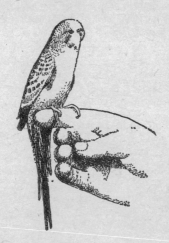

well enough with each other but I had to keep them well away from Pollyo who would have torn them apart.

He was gentle and loving with the dogs, with Rapunzel, with Wanda and with me, but he wouldn't tolerate other birds near him for a minute. He didn't care much for other adults either and I had to warn people who came to the surgery with sick dogs or cats not to be too chummy with him.

He didn't care for strangers who called him Pretty Polly. A bit of a liberty he thought. And if they also poked a finger in his cage—well, that was just asking for it.

Not all visitors to the surgery came with animals. Again and again I would find young women with rather doubtful figures nervously easing themselves into the chair on the other side of my surgery table.

They would then open their handbags, thumb through a wad of notes, and start to tell me about a friend. It was always a friend. This friend, they would say, was in a delicate situation. Her husband, you see, had been overseas for more than a year, and now, somehow, she found she was expecting. If the husband ever found out he would kill the friend. Wasn't there something I could do for her? If I could terminate a pregnancy in a dog or cat, couldn't I see my way clear . . . And the bank notes would rustle.

Money, if they had only known, was no temptation. If they had offered me a square meal for my dogs, though, I might well have been placed in a moral dilemma . . .

One day a very battered Austin, peppered by bullet holes, drew up at the surgery and a woman who was to become one of my closest allies got out, slammed the door and came diffidently inside. Her name was Emily Hill and she was a family doctor with a prosperous practice at Ashford.

Her neighbour's dog, she explained, had been knocked down by a car and its back was broken. She had taken it to two vets already. Both advised putting it to sleep. Could I do anything? Let me have a look at it, I said.

So that evening she was back again bringing with her a little mongrel in great pain. His back was certainly broken. I gave the dog a sedative and slowly, carefully, set the back in plaster.

After three weeks we were thrilled to find that the little dog was getting movement in his legs and only a month later he was able to walk and even run again.

The plaster had to stay on a while longer just to make sure, and at that moment the dog's owners were evacuated and I didn't see it again.

Three whole years later the family came home and called at once on Dr. Hill. The dog bounded in too, full of beans, and Dr. Hill could hardly believe her eyes. The dog's back was *still* in the plaster cast!

"Why on *earth* haven't you taken that plaster off?" she said.

" You mean we *can* take it off?" they said. " We thought it was permanent!"

Dr. Hill set to work on the spot and the three-year-old plaster cast was off at last.

The dog stood and howled. It felt lost without it, naked, defenceless.

" *Cats,*" roared Dr. Hill suddenly, pointing to the door, and the mongrel raced from the room, its worries forgotten.

She was a remarkable woman, Dr. Hill. Indeed she still is. She went right through the First World War as a nurse, usually near the front line, and was shot through the hand in the Serbian campaign. That didn't hold her up for long. After the war she was tempted to become a vet herself, but qualified as a doctor instead.

I asked her about the bullet holes in her car. " Oh, *those,*" she said. " I was machine-gunned by a German fighter while driving through West Wycombe. I was very annoyed. The car was almost new . . ."

That mongrel was the first of a great many animals she brought me. She would bring them in the back of her perforated car from miles around and, if they were well enough, take them back to their homes afterwards. She was a tower of strength to me.

She has retired now but she hasn't changed a bit. Last time I spoke to her she had just returned from a visit to Pakistan. She spoke of it as if she had popped over to Margate for the day.

Her car has changed though. In the new one there isn't a bullet hole to be seen.

To save time I began to hold evening surgery at the house itself, much to the pleasure of one owner of some highly nervous pekes who stepped inside and said " What a wonderful atmosphere!" This wasn't meant as a compliment to us. What she liked was that damned poltergeist.

She was a tiny quiet woman, devoted to her dogs and she frightened my kennel maids out of their wits every time she called. Once inside the house she would go into a trance and, to everyone's amazement, would start to talk in a deep male Negro voice. It really was extraordinary hearing this basso profondo Southern drawl coming from so small a woman. What the voice said was extraordinary too. The lady's Negro spirit contact seemed alarmingly well informed about my past . . .

The spirit wasn't so well informed about the immediate future, however. At any rate he didn't warn me about the dognapping . . .

The dog that was kidnapped was a peke, a friendly little chap who had managed, as dogs sometimes do, to come between husband and wife.

They had quarrelled bitterly over him as well as over other things, and when they got divorced, which, inevitably, they did, the peke was a central issue. Who should get custody of him? That was the problem. In the end the dog went to the wife.

She brought him to me and asked me to guard him with my life. As soon as she had got settled she would come for him. Until then *no one, particularly* her ex-husband, was to take him away.

Two months passed. Then the ex-husband arrived. He had just called, he said casually, for his pekinese.

I said I was terribly sorry but he couldn't have him. "What do you *mean* I can't have him?" he said, furious. "He's *my* dog."

The scene that followed wasn't very pleasant. He got angrier by the minute. He threatened to call the police. He promised to knock my block off. But I was adamant and he left fuming.

A few days later I was coping with a minor crisis on the bank of the lake. A large old raft was permanently moored there. It had been there when we arrived and we regarded it more as a jetty than a raft. It was a shady spot and the dogs liked to lie there when the weather was hot.

That day the mooring rope had finally rotted away and the raft had slowly drifted to the centre of the lake, bearing with it Boozer, Baron and Baroness, three other dachshunds and Rapunzel.

There they sat looking distinctly anxious, with the Khaki Campbells swimming round them, quacking their satisfaction at this turn of events.

While I was organising a pole to drag them back to dry land one of the kennel maids hurried over looking worried.

Had I seen the divorcee's peke? "He's in the paddock," I said. "He's not," she said. And he wasn't. Nor was he anywhere else.

I had a nasty feeling I knew what had happened. I telephoned the police and in half an hour they had news for me. A well-dressed man with a peke under his arm had been seen getting on a train in Feltham station . . .

Now the wife had to be told. She took the news grimly. "Leave this to me," she said.

A few days later she telephoned me again. Her husband had been found, she said. He had handed the peke over to her. There would be no more trouble of *that* kind, she said.

I don't know if there was or not. She didn't entrust me with the little dog again . . .

This was the only dog we ever had stolen, but we did have one or two who ran away. They would be trying to find their way back to their old homes and usually got hopelessly lost. It isn't every dog that is born with the unerring sense of direction of a homing pigeon.

But I had one little dog that did have a remarkable homing instinct.

He was a smooth-haired terrier called Bob and he had been bombed out. His master brought him in and asked me to keep him for the rest of the war. The house had gone, he explained, and he was taking a war job in another town and would be living in digs.

That night Bob got out and we didn't see him for almost a week. Then he turned up again, tired and hungry and ready to settle down.

Neighbours in Sunbury, where his home had been, told me later that they had seen him sniffing round the ruins of his old home. He had found his way there, discovered his master was gone and had come all the way back.

I thought this was an astounding performance.

Bob had been lucky in his master who had obviously earned this kind of devotion. Not all dogs are as fortunate.

Cruelty to animals takes many forms, of course, and

the unhappiest thing about a vet's life is that he sees them all.

One unhappy afternoon a cat with terrible wounds was brought to me. It had been speared with a garden fork by a man who just wanted to spite his wife who loved the cat. I had to put the poor thing out of its misery at once and later, when the man was charged with cruelty, I had to give evidence. He was found guilty and, after being fined the immense sum of ten shillings, left the court, smiling and well pleased.

Luckily, this kind of wanton viciousness is rare. Much more common are stupidity, ignorance, forgetfulness and simple indifference.

In the evacuation of London all four combined to bring fearful suffering to a great many domestic pets. I found myself treating dog after dog suffering from starvation and exposure. They had been tied up in backyards and just left there when their owners shut up their houses and moved to the country.

I was called in to treat one dog that was still alive after three weeks without food. He had been tied to the handle of a backyard door and abandoned without a second thought. He was too far gone and had to be put to sleep.

After incidents like this I would return to Clymping Dene desperately depressed.

There I would be welcomed noisily by Pollyo, lovingly by Wanda, enthusiastically by Boozer, Shush, Baron and Baroness, Angus and Robin, over-enthusiastically by Tasha and fastidiously by Rapunzel.

My mother would have feeding problems to discuss, the kennel maids' crises to report, there would be sick animals to visit and healthy ones to check over. Soon I would be utterly absorbed in my work again and the sordid tragedy of the dog could be pushed to the back of my mind. No one who loved animals could be depressed for long at Clymping Dene.

In the early days of the war my mother's passion for organising and her addiction to Good Works had been completely satisfied by the W.V.S. She threw herself wholeheartedly into the work they did and was rarely at home. It was just like the old days.

But there were now Good Works to be done right in her own back garden and before long the animals of Clymping Dene were absorbing all her time and energy.

Very useful she was too. She was very good at collecting food and almost as good at preparing the big bowls of curious hash that were cooked up in the kennel kitchens to fill two hundred and more hungry animals. She became an expert at making a little go a very long way.

She was on friendly terms with all the dogs, but her love she kept for Fridge, the greyhound, and for the mongrels. One of these was the original shaggy dog, a scruffy little chap called Spats. He looked like a very small Old English sheepdog with white feet and a grey body and my mother and he were always together.

I knew exactly what the attraction was to my mother. Spats represented The Underdog. And underdogs, human and animal, were the abiding passion of her life.

THIRTEEN

The war passed at last. Peace broke out and we celebrated by calling out the hearse for the jolliest journey it was ever likely to make.

We piled into it, my mother, two of the kennel maids, a couple of chums, the undertaker's wife and me, and, with the undertaker at the wheel we bowled off to London.

We parked, I remember, in Grosvenor Street and we then went off for a knees-up in Piccadilly and a riproaring sing-song in Trafalgar Square and up the Mall to Buckingham Palace, swept along by the happiest, most boisterous crowds London has surely ever seen.

It was a wild, glorious binge of a night. The war was over, the killing and the destruction had stopped. We felt light-headed with relief and thankfulness and joy.

I can't remember much about that night except that we lost each other and found each other and lost each other again, that we found our way back to the hearse as dawn was breaking and that we drove back home, quiet, tired and deeply content.

Now the time had come for my great noisy, boisterous family to break-up, each dog and cat returning to its own home. To my astonishment I found that this wasn't going to be easy. We phoned, we wrote, we pleaded, but many owners no longer wanted the pets they had pressed on me with such urgency and gratitude five years before.

Some of the dogs weren't young when they came to me. Now they were five years older and had begun to get a middle-aged spread. Then again the fashion was for smaller animals, for little poodles with fancy clips for toy dogs. Owners had lost interest in the labradors, the dalmatians, the alsatians, that had once been the centre of their lives.

Letter after letter went unanswered. One afternoon I saw the owners of one of my charges passing the surgery door. I had been looking after their big, happy-go-lucky mongrel for almost five years while the husband was in the army and the wife in munitions and, knowing they were together again, I had written to them three times without a reply.

So I called out to them and they stopped.

"Well," I said, "it's nice to see you after all these years. When are you going to collect your dog?"

"Oh that," said the wife, "we don't want him now. You see we're going to buy a Scottie . . ."

And a couple of days later I saw them in the village again. This time they were coaxing a smart little Scottie in a bright tartan coat along the street on the end of a matching tartan lead.

I spent more time than usual with the big old mongrel that night. He was such a dear old fellow. But if his owners wouldn't have him, who would?

Many people did, of course, collect their pets and some of the reunions were very touching. There was the woman who stood with tears in her eyes, holding out her arms towards a handsome little peke who had been with me for three years. He stood watching her, his head slightly on one side, his tail wagging cautiously. He appreciated her obvious goodwill. But who on earth was she? He obviously couldn't remember.

Dogs do have short memories and many of them had forgotten their old masters and their old homes. They are, furthermore, conservative creatures who dislike change. Again and again they plainly showed their reluctance to leave, whining and dragging their feet and looking mournfully over their shoulders as they were led down the drive.

And quite honestly I hated to see them go. Many had been with me for so long that they had become part of my life.

Most of the cats were collected without much prompting from me. In quite a few cases their owners had been killed in the bombing. For these I found new homes.

The horse was collected, so were the parrots and five of the seven tortoises—though they took some finding. Whenever a tortoise owner turned up a search party had to turn out.

Queenie was collected promptly and departed, looking irritated, under the *left* arm of her owner, and Bob, the smooth-haired terrier, recognised his master at once and almost went mad with joy and excitement.

About ten dachshunds were claimed and I must say their owners looked a bit sheepish. The wartime propaganda had worn off quickly. Dachshunds were small enough to be fashionable again and soon they were as popular as they had ever been. It was now the gallant British bulldog's turn to feel the draught. Big, ungainly, chronically short of breath, the bulldog does not fit easily into a small flat or modern semi. The bulldog won the war, but in peacetime it was the chic little dachshund that was in demand.

Fridge, the greyhound, had died late in the war. So had Angus, the west highland white, who caught meningitis, to the distress of Robin, who was heartbroken. I also was very upset.

Pollyo had gone too. One night he was ill. The following morning he was dead. He had caught pneumonia and at his age couldn't fight it. He was almost seventy. I missed him terribly. I had loved that parrot.

Our numbers were going down—but slowly. I now set about finding new homes for the uncollected dogs and cats and all my friends rallied round and helped. Ursula Bloom, who writes splendid magazine articles as well as her books, wrote about my problem several times and offers of homes flowed in from all over the country. Thirty dogs found new homes as a result.

No one would take poor Tasha. No one but my mother wanted Spats or two other mongrels. An easy-going Staffordshire bull-terrier called Mary stayed. So did two alley cats called Ooflang and Carlo, four budgerigars, two tortoises and twenty-four dachshunds, including Boozer, Shush, Baron and Baroness. So did little Robin. So, of course, did Rapunzel and Wanda.

The rest of our family were now widely scattered and, with so few of us left, Clymping Dene was unnaturally quiet. It felt like a school in holiday time, a holiday camp in the winter. None of us seemed at ease.

But I had made my plans for the future. The damp air of the Thames Valley was doing my chest no good and doctors kept telling me so. Get to the coast, they told me. You need sea air.

So I went house hunting in Brighton again. I wanted another Clymping Dene but this time by the sea. I wanted a biggish house that could include my surgery and a large walled garden that could be equipped with the best kennels and the finest cattery in the South of England.

I was given a list of houses to look at. And, miraculously, the first house I looked over was exactly right. The moment I walked through the lich gate I felt I was coming home. I cancelled all the appointments to see other houses. This was it.

It was a sixteenth-century house of great charm, with low gables, small leaded windows, and thick walls heavy with ivy and virginia creeper. The garden took away my breath with its beauty. My heart pounded as I rang the bell and waited to meet the owner.

This was a widow who lived there with her elderly mother and aunt. They were most terribly sorry, they said, but the house was sold. Or almost sold. Nothing was signed but they had given their word. Or almost given their word.

I was nearly overwhelmed by disappointment. I told them how exactly right their house was, that I was a vet and had been hoping to bring sick dogs and cats there to make them well. "But that would be so *right*," said the mother. "The garden would like that very much," said the aunt, " it's already a bird sanctuary." " I think, perhaps, the other gentleman wouldn't mind . . ." said the widow.

And so the house became mine after all.

I hurried home to break the good news to my mother and my sister and then straight away put my Feltham practice and the remainder of my Clymping Dene lease up for sale. I got takers for both almost at once.

There was a lot to do before we could move, but first I called on each of the neighbours whose gardens joined ours, asking if they'd mind if I built kennels. None had any objections and so I went ahead.

The kennels were models of their kind, spacious, comfortable, well heated and with electric light. I put up a sick bay nearby and a whelping pen for mothers and their pups. Then I found a splendid site for the cattery with a tree stump for claw sharpening in the middle of the run.

Again I built more accommodation than I thought I'd ever need. Again I was to be thankful that I'd done so.

The garden was beautiful but it was fantastically overgrown. Trees and bushes hugged the house close, darkening all the windows and the rest was jungle.

The house itself was picturesque but it could hardly have been darker if all the windows had been bricked in. Not only did trees, bushes and creepers hug it close, but all the rooms were painted in the darkest brown.

The hall and the sitting room had huge old fireplaces and every now and then a twig would clatter into the grate. Rooks, building their nests in the friendly old chimneys, were apt to be butter-fingered.

We got to work, cutting back the branches covering the windows, stripping layer after layer of paint away inside and laying bare the most beautifully carved oak panelling. The rooks were dispossessed.

By the time we'd finished the house was light, welcoming and graceful. I felt it had been sleeping for years and we had woken it at last.

I renamed it Dene's Close and, on 13th November, 1946, the furniture vans arrived at Clymping Dene, filled up and set off for the coast.

The furniture was easier to move than the animals. But various friends rallied round and we assembled a little fleet of private cars and one van.

Into these went thirty dogs, five goats, four budgies, three cats, two tortoises, a rather rumpled bantam called Cocky whom I couldn't leave behind and one hugely excited monkey.

We said goodbye to the house. We said goodbye to the gardens, to the deserted cattery, to the empty kennels. We said goodbye to the handful of chickens which were staying behind and to the Khaki Campbells. They went with the lake. We had had our differences, the Khaki Campbells and ourselves, but they were all forgotten. Now we hated to see them pass out of our lives.

Then our little armada of animal-and-bird laden cars set out, winding along the little country roads to join the busy open road to the sea.

FOURTEEN

The journey down was, to put it mildly, eventful.

I had ten dogs in my little car and half way there one of the dachshunds, heavy in whelp, decided that this was the ideal time and place to give birth to her puppies and placidly produced a family of five to the enormous interest of the other passengers. Then we got on our way again. Having set out with ten dogs, I arrived with fifteen. And once installed in her new kennel she went on to produce six more that night.

The other dogs greeted their new garden with ecstasy, bounding across the lawns and chasing each other round the trees and the paddock.

Two of the cats went straight to the cattery, which seemed to meet with their approval, and Rapunzel stalked into the sitting room of the house, found her favourite chair and went to sleep on it. Cocky swaggered in after her and was firmly asked to leave.

The goats, in a bad temper after their journey, were introduced to the goatery and left there to cool off a bit, the tortoises were hibernating and slept through it all, the four budgies, sole survivors of a flight of a hundred, found themselves in a big cage inside the house and made as much noise about it as they could, which was a great deal.

And Wanda loved the house on sight. She explored every nook and cranny—and sixteenth-century houses have crannies and nooks in abundance—scampered round the garden, inspected the kennels and the cattery, peeped into the goatery and retreated hurriedly, and then scrambled on to my shoulder, full of happy noises.

Unfortunately the excitements of the day, combined with the sea air that was to do me so much good, went to the dogs' heads.

They let off steam that night by barking their heads off until four in the morning. They never behaved like this normally. I lay in bed and cursed my luck.

Sure enough next morning an angry neighbour complained and backed his complaint with the threat of legal action.

Next night the dogs slept in the house. I broke up their new runs and had the kennels rebuilt in a different place.

It was a financial body blow. It had cost me several hundred pounds to have kennels built in the first place. Now it cost me several more to have them all pulled down and put up somewhere else.

But I had not time to worry about this or anything else. My plate was put up by the lich gate that first morning and in the afternoon I had my first client.

A tough little man drove up, said his name was Harry and placed in my hands a creature that astonished me. I thought at first it was some species of rat—a rat with matchstick legs, a bulging forehead and pointed ears. It was, he said proudly, a chihuahua.

Chihuahuas have become fashionable since then and can be seen any Sunday morning having a nervous scamper on the lawns of Hove before being scooped up again by their mistresses. But then they were very rare and indeed this was one of the first to be seen in England. I heard afterwards that it had been smuggled in by a Canadian soldier in his kitbag, which it can't have cared for much, and now it caused a sensation wherever it went.

Now people who like chihuahuas like chihuahuas and

people who don't, don't. I'm somewhere in the middle. All I can say is that they aren't my kind of dog. This one was as frail as he looked and needed a lot of attention. But he responded and gradually became perkier and Harry was delighted. So delighted indeed that he declined to pay me in

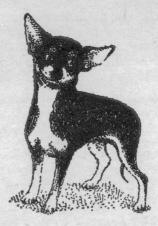

mere money. What, as he so rightly said, is money? Instead he filled the boot of my car with bottles of whisky and gin, with packets of butter, with sugar and tea.

It is hard nowadays to remember just how staggering a payment this was in those days. You just couldn't get riches of this kind. No fee could have been more welcome—until I realised the nature of Harry's business. A few weeks later he came to me with a proposition. The police were beginning to take an unhealthy interest in him, he said. My paddock and cellars were good safe places. Could he store a truckload of crates there until the heat was off? Harry, it seemed, was up to his eyes in the black market. I firmly declined and was deeply grateful that the chihuahua needed no further treatment.

Meanwhile fees of a more orthodox kind were starting to come in. This was just as well. After buying and equipping this house and garden I was broke and having to resite the kennels hadn't helped.

Towards the end of my first week the telephone rang and I found that the multi-millionaire miller, Mr. J. V. Rank was on the line.

"I don't know what's the matter with my dogs," he said. "All I know is that they're all ill. When can you see them?"

"I'll come now," I said.

"Do you know what time it is?" he said.

I did know. It was after 10 p.m. and it was a filthy night.

"The sooner I see them the better," I said.

"Very well," he said, "I have no faith in any treatment, but do what you can."

Now Joseph Rank had one of the finest kennels in the country. He bred wolfhounds and great danes, boxers and wire-haired dachshunds, and his dogs were famous in show rings all over Europe.

The kennels were at Godstone, about an hour's drive away. I arrived about 11 p.m. and was met by Bill Siggars, the kennel manager, who showed me round straight away.

The dogs were in a terrible way. The entire kennel had been swept by a highly contagious streptococcal disease and no dog had escaped. Some were paralysed, others losing their sight. Many were near death.

I set to work on them and by 5 a.m. had done as much as could be done at that stage. I left strict instructions about diet and treatment which Siggars followed to the letter, and that first week I returned every day and frequently after that. All the dogs were well again within the month.

Joseph Rank was, of course, well pleased and I was called in for advice many times in the years that followed.

This was my first major kennel. Others weren't long in following. Indeed, in the years ahead I was to work in most of the winning kennels in Britain.

We had a very bad winter that year. No sooner had the dogs and cats settled in their new homes than the snow started to come down hard.

The garden looked enchanting, the grass, the bushes and the trees all heavy with snow, and the dogs, their kennels snugly heated, seemed to enjoy it.

The cats were a bit disgruntled, though, and so was

Wanda, who sat looking at the snow through the windows, grumbling away.

Like a little girl unable to go out to play, Wanda was bored. So my mother, who always believed the devil would find work for idle hands to do, taught her to knit and to sew.

Wanda was entranced. She did not become the finest seamstress one could meet, but she was certainly one of the most contented. She would sit for hours, making monumental stitches in pieces of cloth with a needle and a piece of bright-coloured wool or pulling the wool laboriously round her knitting needles in a heroic attempt to manage one plain and one pearl.

While she was sewing by the fire I would be trying to get the car out of the garage blocked by snowdrifts, anxious to get to a sick dog at the other side of Sussex, or trying to clear a path to the kennels to get at patients in need of constant attention.

I enjoyed that winter, though, snow and all. My practice was building faster than I dared hope.

I had brought two kennel maids with me from Clymping Dene—Betty Hoxey, who is now a highly successful breeder with her own kennels and a distinguished judge of dachshunds, and Mollie Gingild. As the kennels and the cattery filled my staff grew to four, then to five, then to six.

Soon more than four hundred dogs a month were coming to my surgery. Many came to me as hopeless cases, paralysed, wracked with pain, wasted by disease. I spent many nights sitting up till dawn with desperate cases and sometimes, after a long fight, I would lose a patient. Gloom would fall and a deep depression set in until the next difficult case responded with success. Most, thank God, responded and it was wonderful to see them becoming their old selves again.

Every week, too, there were scores of visits to be made to dogs and cats too sick to be moved. There were the kennels to visit, the farms, stables and piggeries.

I had thought life would be more leisurely now that the war was over.

I was mistaken.

FIFTEEN

While the war lasted I couldn't put my theories about animal feeding into practice. I was only too pleased to get them fed at all.

But now I had my chance. Every dog or cat that came to Dene's Close went straight on to the sort of régime that they should have been on all their lives. They got raw meat and plenty of it, cut into large lumps that they could really get their teeth into. They got raw herring, which dogs as well as cats can learn to love. They got whole grain cereals and wheat germ meal, seaweed powder, parsley and watercress, garlic and cod liver oil and plenty of natural calcium to promote strong bone. One day a week they had a fast—but plenty of honey and water and as much free exercise as possible. Dogs new to this didn't care much for it at first, but soon they came to accept their fast day as a matter of course and were much better for it.

If you keep pets I urge you to feed them like this. In their natural state they would feed themselves properly, catching smaller animals and tearing them with their powerful jaws, swallowing them raw, fur and all. They had no one to cook them breast of chicken in the wilds. They would then go on to find a bountiful supply of all the minerals and vitamins they needed in any wood or meadow, and when they were sick their instincts would lead them to the wild herbs that held the cure.

But fed on the artificial foods of civilisation they sicken. So do we, of course, but that is our look-out. They deserve better.

You had only to look at some of the dogs that came in to know they had been living from table-scraps and cooked mush.

The dogs would be at the same time over-weight and undernourished. Their eyes would lack lustre and their coats would be dull, they would have had breath and skin trouble, quite apart from the more serious disorders that were the cause of the visit. It was remarkable to see how quickly they responded as soon as they were fed properly.

My methods were sometimes attacked by orthodox vets. They called me a crank—well-meaning, of course, and curiously successful, but a crank all the same. I didn't mind this in the least. After all I was seeing my nature cure proving itself every day.

When the snow disappeared and the spring came and the garden sprang to life again I was fascinated to see the dogs foraging for the wild garlic and the parsley that grew like weeds there.

The garden was also rich in witch hazel, which produces one of nature's purest medicines with wonderful purifying and healing powers, and wild elderberries flourished there too. I had learned as a boy how birds ate elderberries to store iron for the hard times in the winter. Now it was interesting to see dogs—particularly sick ones—eating them for just the same reason.

But few people were lucky enough to have herbs and berries growing abundantly right under their windows. So I asked a manufacturing chemist to make up some pills to my prescription.

High on my list were garlic pills. Garlic has been in active use in medicine for more than five thousand years and contains nature's strongest disinfectant. I don't know whether this makes the French a particularly healthy race or not, but I have seen how it destroys bacteria within an animal's system, tones up the lymphatic cells and purifies the blood stream and intestines.

These garlic pills of mine are still used in kennels all over the country.

Then I drew up a prescription for greenleaf pills which are an enormous help for rheumatism and kidney troubles. I fed these to brood bitches, to stud dogs and to puppies and found an immediate improvement in their condition. These, too, went on to the market.

I had rhubarb tablets made up to be taken on the evening before the fast day to help the animals get rid of waste matter, and seaweed powder to give my dogs iron to improve their coats and pep them up generally.

I ordered large quantities of dried parsley and watercress, the richest known source of Vitamin A, and got raspberry leaf tablets made to make whelping easier.

I experimented with elderberries and ordered elderberry pills, strong in natural iron and marvellous for blackening dogs' noses and the rims of their eyes, and devised some nerve pills to quieten dogs with chorea, fits and hysteria, and to steady highly-strung dogs before going into the show-ring.

And because it was hard to get good whole-grain biscuits I made up a cereal I called Naturemeal and had that put on the market too. Then there was Naturebone to give calcium to bitches in whelp and to pups, liver pills and a variety of other products.

I found myself involved in all sorts of tycoon-like activities, attending meetings, signing contracts, agreeing to a percentage on this and a percentage on that. It was all very high-powered stuff.

In fact I made very little money out of it all. These natural supplements to an animal's diet don't cost much and the animal owners don't need large quantities. And the percentages were small.

But the main thing was that they were used up and down the country and still are—and that wherever they are used, dogs and cats are the healthier and happier for it.

And not only dogs and cats . . .

That great actor Robert Donat started calling in for greenleaf pills. He came once a week, collected a packet of them and was on his way. One week I asked him how his dog was doing.

" I don't have a dog," he said. " These are for me . . . They're doing me a power of good."

After that I was astonished and delighted to discover that other people were taking them too.

Charles Hughesden, the millionaire financier, sent his Rolls along to pick up seaweed pills; his wife, Florence Desmond, took greenleaf pills, and so did Elizabeth Allan, the film and television actress. They still take them today. Godfrey Winn said that the seaweed pills kept his figure in trim, and Percy Hoskins, the famous crime reporter, swears by the liver pills. He takes the same dose as for a Great Dane.

They were right, of course. These are all natural cures and are as effective for us as they are for our pets, though I think we'd find Naturemeal a rather sombre breakfast cereal and I certainly don't suggest we should eat our meat raw and in great chunks.

The weekly fast day, though—that I do recommend. You will hate it at first, but your overworked digestive system will love having a regular day off. It will do you the world of good, I assure you.

If you feed yourself wrongly you'll always feel vaguely unwell and you won't look too good either.

The classic example of a wrongly fed dog was Sir Winston Churchill's celebrated brown poodle, Rufus.

Rufus arrived to see me one day on the back seat of a chauffeur-driven car. He was a nice little chap but very spoiled indeed. He was plump and lethargic and his teeth were in an awful state.

"What *has* this dog been eating?" I said.

The chauffeur looked despairingly to the sky.

"Chocolates," he said.

Rufus's trouble was, of course, Sir Winston. He loved the dog. He loved chocolates. So he gave the one to the other. Indeed he gave the dog anything he happened to be eating himself. If Rufus had been a smoker he'd have had the finest Havanas. . . .

Poor Rufus lost most of his teeth that day. I took them out and he was far better and healthier without them.

"Now here is a diet sheet," I said firmly. "Tell Sir Winston it *must* be followed."

"A diet?" said the chauffeur. "For Rufus? You must be joking!"

A similar view was taken by Gilbert Harding.

I had met him several times and knew how much he spoiled Shampoo, his pekinese.

So when he rang up and asked if I would treat the peke I said I would—but only if he would co-operate.

"You must stick to the diet," I said.

Harding rumbled like a volcano about to erupt.

"I don't believe in diets for myself and I don't believe in diets for my dogs," he said. "Good day to you."

So that was that.

SIXTEEN

Late one June evening I was called urgently to some kennels where a number of golden retrievers were seriously ill. They were having fits and were covered with running sores.

The breeder, a brisk no-nonsense sort of a woman, wanted them cured at once and the sickest of them put to sleep. Might as well cut her losses, she said. No point in pouring good money after bad.

I treated each of the sick animals in turn, giving instructions about care and diet as I went along, and then came to the sickest of them all.

"Don't bother about her," said the breeder.

I examined the retriever bitch thoroughly.

"She's in a bad way," I said, "but she deserves a chance. . . ."

"Oh, just put her to sleep," the breeder snapped.

"But we may be able to pull her through," I said.

"Don't waste time," said the breeder. "Put her to sleep and have done with it."

At that I lost my temper.

"Frankly," I said, "I'd rather put you to sleep."

She stormed away and returned with her husband, a peppery man at the best of times.

"How dare you talk to my wife like that?" he shouted.

I told him how I dared. I told him what I thought of him, his wife, and the way they ran their kennels. They gave as good as they got. As shouting matches go it was an all-star spectacular.

It ended with me driving away, as angry as I've ever been. The sick retriever went with me.

That morning my assistant, Diana Abbott, had said, "Don't whatever you do bring another dog back. The kennels are

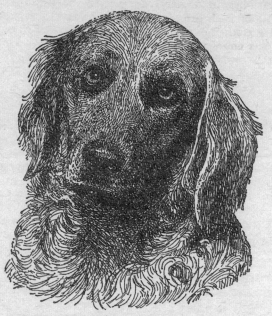

full." So that night the retriever slept in my bedroom.
Next morning I had to leave early for the Cotswolds and
treat kennels there. She came with me in the car, lying beside
me, one heavy paw on my arm. That night she again slept in
my bedroom.

The days passed and treatment and the right diet began to
do their work. Slowly at first, then in leaps and bounds, she
got better and better. Her coat grew again, thick, shining and
golden. Her eyes brightened, her energy flooded back.

This, then, was Jackie, who hardly ever left my side for
the next ten and a half years.

She became the spirit of Dene's Close. She had an extraordinary smile and quite naturally took charge of all the
other dogs, looking after them and calming them when they
were nervous. She met all visitors at the lich gate and led
them to the surgery and I only once saw her lose her temper.

I had put her in for a Champion Dog Show and she

covered herself in glory and won all classes. But in the middle of it all she suddenly stiffened, bared her teeth and gave a ferocious growl. From this sloppy, over-affectionate dog this was unbelievable. Then I saw what she had seen—her previous owner. Elephants aren't the only creatures with memories.

Wanda, Rapunzel, Boozer and Cocky all took to Jackie at once, accepting her natural, gentle, unassertive authority and so did newcomers to the house. Like Peter Whistle.

Peter Whistle was a mynah bird, a glossy little black chap with a bright yellow beak. A client brought him in for treatment and then asked if I'd like to keep him. Mynah birds, he said, tended to get above themselves. Never stopping *talking,* he said. And cheeky with it.

So Peter Whistle stayed. He was certainly a phenomenal talker, and if you said "Oh, shut up, Peter!" he would say "Oh, shut up, Peter," back in exactly the tone you had used.

In time he learned to imitate my voice so uncannily well that people, hearing him chatting away in another room, would be astounded to see me in the far reaches of the garden. This could be very embarrassing. People who called when I was away would be just about to leave when Peter would pipe up in the next room. "I thought you said Mr. Lloyd-Jones was out," they would say coldly to my assistant. "Please tell him I'm here."

"That's only Peter Whistle," she would say, embarrassed. "*Shut up, Peter.*"

"*Shut up, Peter,*" he would shout back.

Pandora was a Siamese cat who thought she was a dachshund.

She came to me extremely sick, sent by people I didn't know and couldn't trace. Later I found that a judge had given her to his son and daughter-in-law. They had gone off on holiday, leaving the poor thing locked in an expensive flat in Belgravia with a few bottles of milk with the tops off and some opened tins of cat food. They were away for weeks and when the cat was found at last she was in a pitiful state.

When she came to see me she was so ill that for four weeks she would neither eat nor drink. The stamina of animals can

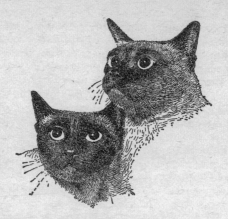

be astonishing. She became a skeleton, poor creature, unable to move but she was still alive.

We gave her crushed garlic, honey and water, as much sun as possible and a lot of love and very, very slowly she began to take an interest in life again. All her life she had been cooped up in a small flat and had seen few, if any, dogs before. Now she attached herself to a paralysed dachshund and shared his basket and it was touching to see the love these two sick animals had for each other.

The owners never got in touch with me again, thinking, no doubt, she was dead, and so she stayed. She grew into a sweet, lovely creature but to the end of her life she clearly believed she was a dachshund herself and only seemed really happy with dachshunds round her. We never had the heart to tell her . . .

Soon afterwards two more Siamese cats joined us. Their names were John and Josephine. They came to me after the divorce of their owners. They had gone with the wife who adored them—but she had had to go back to work and couldn't look after them. She asked if I would keep them for the time being, I agreed, and they duly arrived. Before she left their owner gave elaborate instructions about food and exercise to the kennel maid and left with words that became famous at Dene's. "They'll be all right," she said, "just as long as they never meet a dog. . . ."

Well, of course you couldn't be at Dene's Close for five minutes without meeting dogs, much to the pleasure of John and Josephine. They were, in fact, more like dogs than cats. They played with the dogs for hour after hour and at night they slept in their kennels.

I had both for the rest of their lives—John for nine years and Josephine for twelve. They were always together but they were, as actresses say to airport reporters, just good friends.

Where love was concerned Josephine ignored poor John completely. She preferred a neighbouring ginger tom whom we all called Ginger Rogers. She produced litter after litter—and always the father was Ginger. I was always hoping for at least one pure-bred Siamese litter, if only as a boost for John's ego, but it was Ginger who had the sex-appeal.

Every now and then Josephine got asthma—sometimes quite badly. She would wheeze away and go very thin and look quite dreadful. I would be able to ease the discomfort, but asthma is a tricky thing to deal with and Josephine had these attacks all her life.

Just before Christmas one year a school teacher who lived nearby called in for some advice. She had found this pathetic Siamese cat, she said, absolutely starving. She seemed to be in a very bad way. What should she do? I gave her advice about feeding the cat up and putting it back into condition with powders and vitamins and she went her way.

A few days later she was back to borrow a cat basket. She was going to Exeter for Christmas, she said, and she would have to take the poor cat with her.

That night I couldn't find Josephine anywhere. She had been in and out of the surgery wheezing away with asthma all morning, but no one had seen her since.

Suddenly the penny dropped. The teacher's starved Siamese was asthmatic Josephine, who had got on to a good thing. She had eaten her usual hearty dinner at Dene's and had popped out for another hearty meal across the garden . . .

I rang the teacher at once. Too late. She had already left for Exeter, taking Josephine with her. I was a bit worried about Josephine's asthma and anyway we wanted her home for Christmas, so I got the teacher's holiday address and rang her up.

"You know that half-starved Siamese?" I said. "Well, her name is Josephine and she belongs to me. Could I have her back, please?"

Josephine arrived back next day. We put the basket on the surgery table, opened it and out she jumped looking marvellous. Her asthma had passed and she was sleek and handsome and delighted to be home again. She purred and rubbed herself against us, was unusually affectionate to John and then made for the kennels to sleep it off.

Then a second golden retriever arrived. I had been to a cocktail party in London and the owner of the flat said her dog was ill in the next room. So, taking my drink with me, I had a look.

Cleo was lying on the bed, very sick indeed. She had enteritis. I couldn't do anything there so when I left I took her with me.

I said I couldn't keep her more than five days as it was Christmas and the kennels were full and I tried to give the staff a little time off. Not that they ever got much time off at Christmas or any other time. They were wonderful people.

Five days got her over her immediate crisis and she returned to London on Christmas Day very much better. But after a few weeks in London she became dull and lethargic and her owner brought her back again. "She's miserable in London," she said. "Could she stay here a while?" She stayed for nine years.

She completely lost her London lethargy, though she could be a bit slow at times. When she was in whelp she enjoyed her pregnancy enormously and in fact was eight days overdue. She was *enormous* and would sit smiling quietly to herself while we all worried ourselves silly.

At last she produced eleven pups—one of the best golden retriever litters I've known.

Cocky grew more cocky daily and hated to be left out of things. I had a large dog bed with a spring mattress in the sitting room and here Wanda, Boozer and Rapunzel liked to sleep, all snuggling up to each other. Cocky would stalk in and jump in among them, pushing and shoving to get a warm place.

One night all four were quietly snoozing there before a blazing log fire. My mother was sitting knitting. I was talking to some friends. Suddenly a door banged loudly and Cocky shot up the chimney.

It all happened so quickly that none of us was sure what was going on. There was a squawk from the chimney and a shower of soot and poor Cocky emerged. He was black. He was scorched and shaken. And every feather had been singed off.

I dabbed him with oil to protect his skin and for days he sulked. He wasn't hurt physically, but his pride was deeply wounded. It took three months for the feathers to grow back.

But long before then Cocky was as cocky as ever, stalking about the house and the garden and making sure that no one was in any doubt about who ruled the roost at Dene's Close.

It was about this time that Lady Millicent Taylour, the daughter of Rose, Marchioness of Headfort, brought me her mother's dachshund, Max.

Max, she said, had a very serious complaint. He was over-sexed. Could I please do something to damp his ardour?

Well, indeed I could. I recommended the remedy that has damped male ardour since time began. I found him a wife.

Lady Headfort warmly approved of my suggested treatment, invited me to dinner, and soon I felt I'd known her all my life.

In her youth she had been the famous Gaiety Girl, Rosie Boote, and she had been a great beauty all her life. Even when she reached her seventies she remained a dazzlingly elegant woman.

The wife I chose for Max was a pretty dachshund called Sari, one of Boozer's many daughters—who had already wet-nursed a large litter of pekes. She brought them up beautifully, showing them great love and care.

She and Max took at once to each other and she bore him a fine litter of six. Again she brought up the puppies with loving care. Lady Headfort came down and chose one of the pups—picking, inevitably, the smallest, prettiest and most endearing.

This is always a temptation for tender-hearted women and it is usually a great mistake. The best puppy is the one that bounds forward, wagging its tail and trying to lick your hand. The shy, undersized, appealing fellow who sits in the far corner and just looks at you is the runt of the litter and will probably never be as healthy or as robust as its more extrovert brothers and sisters.

But Lady Headfort was lucky with her pup, who grew up to be very handsome and affectionate. Max outlived him, though. He is still alive—indeed he visited me only the other day with Miss Ferguson, who was Lady Headfort's personal maid for fifty-four years. He is a stately old gentleman now, going grey at the muzzle and, alas, without a tooth in his head.

Lady Headfort thought that everyone should have a dog and gave Cropper, her butler, a fine boxer called Buffer. Buffer too became a patient of mine and, though the dog is dead now, Cropper still comes to see us once a year. He is with Lady Headfort's son now, still butling. Indeed I have never seen anyone butle better.

The kennels and the cattery were intended, and were largely kept, for sick animals. Occasionally, though, I'd be talked into taking in a dog to look after it while its owners were on holiday.

One such dog gave me a very nasty three days. He was a fine golden cocker who watched his owners leaving for their holiday in France with apparent goodwill and seemed to settle down well.

The minute he was left alone he started his great bid for freedom. He bit his way out of his run, leapt over a seven-foot wall and was away.

We discovered he was gone early next morning, at once reported it to the police and started searching the district ourselves.

There wasn't a sign of him anywhere. His owner's neighbours kept a sharp lookout for him too in case he had made for home. No luck.

There was nothing for it. His owners must be told. So I

sent them a wire. They at once packed and caught the next plane back to London. They drove straight home, half expecting to see him waiting on their doorstep. He wasn't though. He was waiting on mine. At almost the very minute his owners opened their front door, he turned up at Dene's Close looking cheerful, healthy and totally unrepentant.

He had been gone for three days—just where he had been no one ever found out. I telephoned his owners at once, of course, and they received my call with what you might well call mixed emotions. They were pleased he was back of course. But they weren't too pleased to have cut their holiday short after only two days—and to no purpose.

They spent the rest of that holiday at home. And next year, I noticed, they made other arrangements.

Much the same thing happened when Mary Kessell, the artist, sent her dachshund Ricky to me for treatment.

He was let out with the other dachshunds into the gardens in the evening for their last calls and when the dogs came in one of them was missing. It was Ricky . . .

We searched high and low, but there wasn't a trace of him. I passed a sleepless night and next morning telephoned Miss Kessell to break the news. She came down at once and arrived to find Ricky, happy and carefree, and me very red-faced.

Ricky had turned up minutes beforehand, perfectly happy and carefree. The night before he had spent his time in the garden digging himself a beautiful tunnel. Once well under he had curled up and gone peacefully to sleep.

Vets find themselves with some curious telephone calls to make. For instance I remember one very embarrassing call that came my way. I had to ring up a very proper, high-minded lady and tell her that her spaniel dog wasn't a spaniel dog any more. It was now a spaniel bitch. It had, during its stay in my kennels, changed sex.

She was furious. "Impossible!" she cried. Then, "Are you *sure*?" Then. "It's all your fault. You've ruined it's life. *I'll sue*!"

She didn't sue, though. If she had she'd have lost her case. Dogs, like all other animals, are by no means all sexually "normal." And sex changes happen, as in human beings, from time to time.

I have personally known of six such cases in my career as a vet. Dogs become bitches, and though they cannot bear puppies, certainly often have milk in their teats. I have never known a case of a bitch becoming a dog.

With human beings this is always a personal tragedy which deserves our sympathy. But no sympathy is needed for dogs in this predicament. They get along perfectly happily in their new sex. It is the owners that get upset.

SEVENTEEN

Sick animals would arrive at Dene's Close at all hours of the day and night. Animals, like their owners, can't always be ill conveniently between 9 a.m. and 5 p.m. and their litters, again like those of their mistresses, have a way of arriving at 3 a.m.

So an uninterrupted night's sleep became a luxury and a long lie-in in the morning something that just never happened. Every day began at 6 a.m. Animals, sick or well, are early risers.

Any day might bring all manner of small animals and birds for treatment.

One afternoon a tortoise arrived with a broken jaw. He had tangled with a motor mower in Sir Colin Anderson's magnificent garden in Hampstead and I had to pin his jaw with wire and feed him with crushed lettuce and vitamins from a fountain-pen filler. He was a pleasant patient fellow, who became extraordinarily friendly and tame. He stayed on too after he was well and made his home in my garden.

He would plonk himself on my chest when I was sunbathing and would go charging off after other tortoises throughout the mating season. We would hear him making violent love to them—clank, clank, clank. Tortoise shells don't make for discreet relationships. Clank, clank. In the end he died of making love. After a particularly noisy night we found him dead on the lawn. His heart had given out. Even a tortoise can have too much of a good thing.

There were other patients who would have been happy to stay too, but they wouldn't have fitted so easily into the family.

Take George, the Largest Porcupine in Captivity. This is what Brighton Zoo said he was and they may have been right. He certainly was a big porcupine. One day he escaped from his cage and, in doing so, damaged his nose. Two keepers chased after him and naturally he whirled round and shot a quiverful of quills with deadly accuracy into their legs. Off they went to hospital and the zoo called me in.

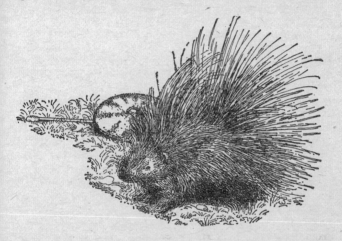

Diana Abbott and I found George entangled in the wire netting of a disused tennis court. He was frightened, edgy, in pain and ready to give battle.

Helped by a long stick and a lot of luck we managed to coax him into a box and whisk him off to Dene's Close. Then, of course, our problems had just begun.

The porcupine's nose was lacerated and he wasn't letting anyone near it. So he became the only patient I ever had to approach from behind a dustbin lid. I held it up like a gladiator's shield in one hand, a long stick with cotton-wool soaked in liquid garlic, nature's disinfectant, in the other, edging nearer and nearer. George watched warily. Every time he rattled his quills in warning I would jump out of the way. One quiverful of quills narrowly missed me, rattling on the dustbin lid and making me feel like a medieval knight.

Eventually, with lots of time and patience, I got near enough and, somehow managed to clean up the wound. The worst was over. After that he didn't mind so much and as the days went by he got to like us. He would watch out for our coming and give little grunts of welcome. And by the time he got back to the zoo he was literally eating out of our hands.

Then there were the wolves. There were four of them in the zoo and they all caught a kind of wolvine distemper.

I treated them, installed them in a kennel in my isolation ward, did my rounds and went to bed. I was awakened by frightening screams from one of the kennel maids. It had been her day off and, returning late, she had looked into the kennels to see how her patients were. She walked in, expecting friendly dogs, and was petrified to find herself facing a wolf pack. She fled and so did the wolves.

The rest of the night was chaotic, but for the wolves a great spree.

They broke into the chicken farm next door and rampaged among them, enjoying an orgy of slaughter and terror. Dachshunds got in to join in the fun, and at the end of it all I was left to foot the bill for the slaughtered chickens.

I've always advocated natural feeding for wolves as much as anyone else. But my neighbours' chickens weren't exactly what I had in mind.

One of the wolves, more ambitious than the rest, came to a violent end that night. Leaving his companions to the chickens, he set off in the direction of London, where, as is well known, the pickings are easier for a wolf of daring and resource.

Alas, he met a taxi head-on in the London Road and was killed outright. The taxi driver, thinking he had hit an alsatian of some kind, must have been astounded to find he had run over a Canadian timber wolf in the heart of Sussex.

Only once did I have a patient too big to come to me. This was a fine Indian elephant who lived in Dublin Zoo.

The superintendent wrote to say that the elephant had a puzzling ailment and would I look in to see her. I'd never treated an elephant before but I was certainly game. I packed my bags and left for Eire.

I found the elephant in a sorry state. Her thick, soft skin was hardening like cement. So there she was, towering above me, slowly turned, so it seemed, to stone.

Among her troubles, apparently, was a serious vitamin

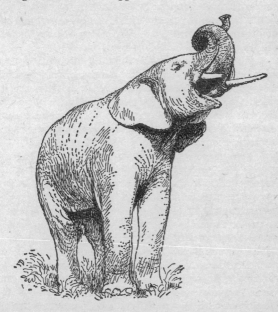

deficiency and I did what I could on the spot to ease the discomfort and told them how they could put the deficiency right. She also really needed an enema, but I rather think I funked that . . .

Before I left again for England and animals of more modest size, the curator took me into the reptile house and gave me one of the more nerve-wracking ten minutes of my life.

I had never met a big snake before—had never much wanted to, actually—but now I found myself surrounded by them. This man was quite wonderful in handling them, picking up pythons and enormous boa constrictors, quietly and without any fuss.

He must have supposed that I was used to snakes as well, because when a huge constrictor slid off him and started to coil itself round me he made no attempt to stop it. I was very frightened indeed, but at the same time I remember how surprised I was to find it warm and dry, not, as I had always imagined, cold and clammy.

There was a crowd of onlookers on the other side of the glass partition, so I put on as brave a face as possible. It's hard to be nonchalant while wearing a very large snake, but I tried. And then, just as I was thinking that I'd had enough, a keeper put his head round the door and told the curator he was wanted on the telephone. "A call from America," he said, laying it on a bit thick.

This was clearly an old gag, a practical joke played on unwary visitors to reptile houses down the ages, but this didn't occur to me till later.

All I knew was I was suddenly alone, alone except for a large and very probably hungry snake which was twined around my neck. It was terribly heavy and I could feel its muscles contracting and relaxing. I tried to loosen its hold, but this only seemed to make it fasten itself more firmly.

So I stood there for what seemed an age, keeping as still as I could and keeping my mind on pleasant things, like vats of boiling oil for humorous reptile keepers.

They rescued me at last and I got back to England, untrampled by sick elephants and undigested by big snakes, to face more mundane occupational hazards.

I hadn't enjoyed my unwilling snake-charming act but I had reason to be grateful for it. Only a few weeks later I found, to my surprise, that my patients included a cobra.

I was called urgently to a small terrace house in Brighton by a man who said that one of his pets had been badly bitten.

He took me at once into the living-room. "This," he said opening the door, " is my snake pit."

There was no furniture in the room. Instead the floor was divided up into five compartments and in each was a snake. Two were cobras, one was a python. I couldn't identify the other two, but they looked a little too lively for my comfort.

"This is the one that's hurt," said the man, picking up one of the cobras and handling it tenderly. It had a fairly deep wound, inflicted, said the man, by one of the other snakes.

I knew nothing about snakes and said so. But the creature clearly needed treatment. So I decided to proceed as if it was a dog.

While he held the snake I cleaned the wound and dressed it, said briskly "Bring him along to the surgery tomorrow," and was on my way.

He came next day, the cobra in a zip-up hold-all, and returned regularly until the wound had healed. His conversation was of nothing but his snakes. He was a working man with a modest wage and his snakes absorbed every penny he could save. He was at that moment saving up for a sixth. "What about your wife," I asked him once, "does she like snakes?"

"Not much," he said.

I must say that the cobra was always very docile when it came to see me, which is more than I can say for some of the dogs.

In fact in all my years as a vet I was never bitten once by a patient, but I sometimes marvel at this when I remember some of the patients I had.

Some owners were actually proud of their dog's uncertain tempers. "You'll be lucky if you get near *him*!" they would say in a satisfied way and they would look taken aback when the dog stopped growling and snapping and stood quietly for examination and treatment.

Alsatians, more than any other breed except perhaps Dobermann Pinschers, have an unenviable reputation. "You can never trust them," people say.

In fact if they are properly trained alsatians are utterly trustworthy. They are a splendid breed—strong, intelligent and affectionate, but it is imperative that their owners must show strength, intelligence and affection too.

The most dangerous dog I ever met was an alsatian brought to me by a man who lived with it in a tiny cottage on the downs. The dog had no training at all and had been allowed to run wild. He had, said the owner as if boasting, already bitten three people and I could tell by the look in the dog's eye that he had a fourth in mind.

He didn't get his teeth into me, though, but he tried. I had to operate on his rear leg, which was very sore for a few days afterwards. This didn't improve his temper and every time I dressed it he had a go at me.

"He's a hard case, he is," his owner would say, grinning triumphantly. It wasn't the dog who was the hard case. It was the man.

Not long afterwards a waiter from one of the big hotels on the front arrived at the surgery with a massive dog on a heavy chain. The animal was half bull mastiff, half labrador, and the little waiter was obviously scared to death of him.

"I want you to bump him off," he said.

"You want me to *what*!" I said, glaring.

"Bump him off," said the waiter. "Do him in. My landlady won't have him in the house. Anyway, he bites . . ."

The waiter obviously couldn't cope, so he went his way leaving his strong and unruly dog with me. He was a handful, certainly. For the first few days he wouldn't let anyone near him. But I persevered, and he soon came to realise that I wasn't afraid of him and would stand no nonsense. With firmness, patience and a lot of affection I taught him to sit, to heel, to stop on command, and in a month or two he was a beautifully mannered dog who could be taken anywhere.

Like all properly trained dogs he was a lot happier too, and when he finally left, to work as a guard dog on a small-holding, we were all sorry to see him go.

Then there was the chow, owned by the popular violinist Reg Leopold. The chow had been trained and was in a beautiful condition—but chows are one-man dogs. They don't take to just anyone and you'd be wise not to be too familiar if you meet a strange chow coming down the road.

This chow needed his teeth scaling. Now no one likes going to dentists, but I must say Mrs. Leopold's chow took it bravely, didn't complain once.

Afterwards I heard why the dog's teeth had needed scaling so badly.

"We've been trying to get them done for ages," said the girl who brought him. "But no one dared do it . . ."

If I'd known this before I started I might have had second thoughts myself.

Chows need a firm hand. But then so do all dogs in varying degrees. However small a dog is he can make a terrible nuisance of himself if he is given all his own way.

Big or small, pedigree or mongrel, all dogs *must* have lessons in how to behave.

They must be taught to walk quietly at your side, to stop on command, to sit on command, to come when they are called. Begin teaching them when they are three months old. Take them out on a choker lead, use simple words of command and make them obey you. When you say sit, make them sit, when you say stop, make them stop. Repeat the exercises over and over again and give them tremendous praise when they do as they are told. Dogs are intelligent creatures. They'll soon catch on.

And for the rest of their lives they will be safe in traffic, well-mannered in other people's houses and relaxing company wherever you are.

This kind of elementary training is more for the dog's benefit than your own convenience. If all dogs are equal the well-trained well-behaved dog is more equal than others.

EIGHTEEN

The Emperor Caligula made his horse a Senator and everyone was properly scandalised. Well he was a *Roman*, you see. Had he been an Englishman no one would have been at all surprised.

All over the world stories are told of the eccentric English and their dotty devotion to animals. I'm English myself and I've spent a lifetime with animals and their English owners. And I'd say that our reputation for dottiness is fully justified.

Almost every day I see a splendid old lady wheeling a twin pram across the road and on to the lawns under my windows.

Strangers peer into the pram, ready to smile at the twins inside. Instead they find two little pekes. Once safely on to the grass, the old lady lifts the dogs out and they run for miles. When they at last return they are popped back into the pram and are wheeled home again.

During the war, I used to treat a big black poodle called Fifi. She was a very grand lady who arrived in state, sitting with royal dignity in a sidecar of a bicycle ridden by her mistress. This lady's life revolved round Fifi to the complete exclusion of her husband. During the war the poor man was even obliged to give up his entire meat ration to this fastidious dog. The war, said her mistress, wasn't *Fifi*'s fault.

The husband was a senior civil servant with a high income, which was just as well because Fifi had expensive tastes. Eventually one flat was no longer enough. The flat next door had to be bought as well because, as his wife explained, Fifi *had* to have her own bathroom and bedroom.

The time came when the poor man had had enough. It was either the poodle, he said, or him. Without the smallest hesitation she chose the poodle and he went quietly out of both their lives.

Poodles do seem to have a curious effect on perfectly sensible women.

I had agreed to take one poodle for a week while her owner was away and the little bitch arrived wearing a blue bow with a matching blue collar. Her mistress then handed me a box and a list. The box contained six more coloured bows and six more matching collars. The list showed which colour must be worn on each day.

Then there was the lady who lived in a very large house in Surrey surrounded by the most glorious grounds. It had once been a lovely mansion but now the dogs had simply taken over and the place was going to wrack and ruin.

There were dogs in every room, dogs in all the outhouses and garages, dogs all over the grounds. When they were hungry they just wandered into the kitchen and tore a bit off the dead sheep that was left for them on the floor. The carcase stayed there until it was eaten, and in the summer the smell and the flies met you as you went in the front door.

Puppies were born in whatever place took the mother's

fancy—in one of the baths, in the butler's pantry, even, in one case, in the Rolls Royce.

The Rolls, indeed, was kept almost solely for the dogs, who were taken out in it in relays every day, and I once saw the owner cleaning out the kennels wearing a silver mink.

This lady thought she had created a paradise for her dogs, but of course she had done nothing of the kind. Many of them were in a terrible condition and my heart sank as the day for my regular visit approached. For one thing it sometimes took my assistant and me from nine in the morning to nine at night to *find* all the dogs and to discover how many needed treatment.

Another of my clients, who lived in a beautiful house in Sussex, was the most extreme kind of vegetarian. I'm a vegetarian myself, but I was always astonished at the lengths one can go to.

Nothing made from leather was allowed in the house. Her shoes, which she made herself, were usually canvas. Fur of any kind, of course, was banned. She even made her own make-up to ensure no animal fats were used.

I once went to dinner there and when we went into the dining room I congratulated her on the charming table decoration. Before each of our plates was a bowl of nasturtiums and they looked very pretty. We sat down and. to my deep embarrassment, I discovered that the flowers were the first course. Carefully following our hostess we dipped each flower into a dressing and solemnly ate it.

This lady had five pomeranians. They, too, had to be vegetarian.

Now this, I think, is very unfair. You have only to look at a dog's teeth and the structure of his jaw to know that this is a carnivorous animal who *needs* meat.

The pomeranians ate their vegetarian meals readily enough and when they were in my kennels for treatment their mistress would visit them with fresh grapes as a special treat which they would eat with pleasure.

But fruit and vegetables alone clearly didn't suit them. They were listless dogs with indifferent coats and dull eyes. But I could never persuade their mistress to change their diets.

Another owner was a very pleasant but nervous woman who lived in a very large house in its own grounds with only three dogs for company—a chow, an airedale and a mongrel called Bonzo.

She was terrified of burglars and so always kept her dining table laid for fourteen people and lights on all over the house to give the impression that the place was well occupied.

Her one little weakness was drink. Every now and then she would treat herself to the original lost weekend and pass out completely. One morning I was told that no one had seen her for three or four days. I was worried both about her and about the dogs who were inside the house too and making a lot of noise. So I broke in.

The dogs were ravenous—and their mistress was dead to the world, drunk as a lord.

When she came to she discovered that a pair of very valuable diamond earrings was missing. Sensation. No one leave the room. Now, sir, where were you on the night of the ninth. Everyone was under suspicion, particularly Bonzo. He had been, we thought, acting most suspiciously and his alibis just didn't hold water.

Bonzo was indeed the culprit. He had swallowed both the earrings. In the fullness of time they were recovered through the normal channels and next time I went to the house the earrings were once again glittering in the lady's ears.

Most of my clients were very kindly, agreeable people. But not all. Occasionally I would meet someone who was very hard to like.

There was a rich young woman in Worcester who had set her heart on becoming a successful dachshund breeder. She travelled all over the country paying exorbitant prices for dachshunds until eventually she had built up quite a large pack.

I used to make a monthly visit to check the kennel over, but in fact she bred very little. There was always some trouble with the dogs and bitches and they were as unhappy a pack of dogs as I have met. Even the house dogs were miserable and seemed to spend much of their time tied up to pieces of furniture.

There was something very unlikeable about this girl, though for a long time I couldn't say what it was. Then one day Diana and I were paying our usual visit when we noticed some goat kids in a paddock. It was a bright windy day and they looked lovely.

We admired them for a while and then went on to the pig-sties, where part of the pack was kept, and started work. After about ten minutes a terrible sound came from the paddock, a yelping and screaming that raised the hair on the back of the neck. We ran out to see what on earth was happening and there were twelve of the dachshunds ferociously attacking two of the kids, tearing them to pieces in front of our eyes.

We raced over and dragged them away—and found we were being watched with some amusement by the girl. "Leave them to it," she said. "That's what the kids are for. The dogs are enjoying themselves."

I was so angry I could hardly speak. The kids, the girl went on, were bred for just this purpose. They afforded the dachshunds both food and sport at very little cost. I always advocated natural feeding, she said. What could be more natural than dogs hunting their food in a pack.

I almost exploded. I don't think I've ever been so rude to a woman before or since and the minute I got away from that hateful place I reported her to the R.S.P.C.A. and the police.

I heard later she had been prosecuted and fined. A fine would make no impression on someone as rich as she was. But perhaps being taken to court may have taught her some sense, if not some humanity. I never went near her again.

A delightful and very rich couple on the Isle of Wight kept tiny Shetland ponies and huge Irish wolfhounds. The hounds towered over the ponies, a sight to shock any passing horse.

One of the wolfhounds—a dog called, perversely enough, Annie—had a recurring form of enteritis and I got used to the urgent summonses from her owners. "Please will you come at once," they would say on the phone. "Charter a plane . . ."

So charter a plane I did again and again, arriving there in a couple of hours and getting back home in time for supper. On one occasion the airport had hired out all its small passenger planes. "You can have an old bomber," they said facetiously. I rang the Isle of Wight and told them the news. "Charter the bomber then," they said. So I found myself all alone in that cavernous interior, droning towards the Isle of Wight to treat a sick dog called Annie. No bomber ever made so peaceful a journey.

Some clients had no sense whatever of time. So they would ring up at all hours of the nights, just for a chat about their animals.

If the telephone went at 4 a.m. I would know just who it would be. Frances Day. She was then at the height of her brilliant career and, as her cabaret would finish in the early hours of the morning, 4 a.m. was merely early evening to her. "It's me," she would say gaily. "I just wanted to enquire about my little Dunham." Little Dunham, I should add, was a huge boxer, one of the biggest I have known.

Actresses aren't the only people without any sense of time. I tried to stop people bringing their dogs to me in the middle of the night, but how can you say no to a distressed woman with a sick animal? How can you say no to a determined woman dog-owner whether her animal is sick or not?

One middle-of-the-night visitor was a breeder from the north who had imported two Rhodesian ridgebacks—the first in the country, she claimed. She mated them successfully and asked if the pups could be born at Dene's. Regretfully I had to say no. The kennels were full.

Late one afternoon she rang me to say that the bitch's labour had begun and that she was on her way. "I'm sorry," I said, "there's no room."

An hour later she rang again. She was ringing from a phone box on the A.1, she said. The bitch was all right so far.

"She can't come *here*!" I said.

Two hours passed and again the phone went. She was two hours nearer, she said, but the bitch had been sick. What should she do? "Go *home* again," I said. No wonder the bitch was sick, making such a long car journey at such a time in her life.

But so it went on throughout the evening, phone calls every two hours, each of them nearer and nearer.

At midnight I put the lights out and went to bed. And at 2 a.m. there was a banging on the door. They had arrived. The owner demanded hot drinks for herself and the chauffeur and then went to sleep on the sitting-room settee while I stayed up with the expectant mother.

The birth was perfectly easy and straightforward and the puppies were healthy and attractive. One, she said, was to be offered to the Queen.

Owner, chauffeur, ridgeback and puppies spent most of the following day in bed and left late in the afternoon on the long drive home.

I must say I admired her determination.

A great many dogs enjoy a beer. Elizabeth Allan had a snow-white bull-terrier called Emily who insisted on her daily pint. If Miss Allan didn't feel like going out, Emily would walk round to the local on her own. I once asked the barman at the pub if Miss Allan had been in that evening. "No," he said, "but Emily was in half an hour ago."

Emily is here no more and her place has been taken by a labrador called Daisy. She has a Guinness a day.

Beer does them little harm actually—malt is a natural food —but all hard-drinking dogs had to become teetotal at Dene's Close.

Denise Robins, the romantic novelist, was deeply devoted to an Australian terrier called Dingo and later to a charming griffon called Gaston.

Once when Dingo was shockingly mauled by a boxer she sent me an urgent telegram to Paris, where I was on holiday, and I flew back to operate. And later, when Gaston disappeared from home, she hired a helicopter to search for him. It criss-crossed the whole of the Ashdown Forest—but not a sign of little Gaston. At last, a week later, when Miss Robins was almost distracted with worry, he was found in a garden twenty-five miles away, emaciated, exhausted but overjoyed to be reunited with her.

With some people ordinary affection for an animal can develop into an obsession. This is not a happy thing to see.

It happened to a very old friend of mine, a man I first

knew before the war. He was happy and gregarious with a tremendous zest for life.

I didn't see him for a few years and then he brought a dog to me for treatment. An alsatian.

The war was over now and he was a Colonel and changed beyond belief. He looked old and ill and melancholy. His old *joie de vivre* had gone entirely.

He talked about his dog—and I understood the change in him.

He had been in command of the troops that first entered Dachau concentration camp, he said. The camp was guarded by ferocious alsatians trained to kill. As a last desperate stroke the dog handlers had released the dogs and, as one alsatian had leaped for him, he had shot its German master dead.

The alsatian had been captured and the Colonel had kept it. He couldn't bring himself to speak of the horrors of the camp itself, but they had almost destroyed him. What had kept him sane was the dog.

The animal was vicious, violent and tried to attack every man it saw in British uniform. For the first few days the Colonel had to keep him chained and muzzled. He would not forget that he had shot down the dog's master and became determined to take his place in the dog's affections. He spent hours pacifying him, talking to him, coaxing him, trying to ease away the hate that had been bred into him.

When the Colonel returned to England the dog came with him—no muzzle now and no chain but walking freely and naturally at his new officer's side.

The dog went into quarantine and the Colonel, now demobbed, bought a house near the quarantine kennels so that he and his wife could visit him every day.

At the end of six months the dog was released and from that moment he and the Colonel were inseparable.

The attachment to the dog was such that there was little affection left over for the wife.

They had been one of the happiest couples I had known. Now they divorced and my friend hardly seemed to notice.

He was content enough in his new, sombre way until the

alsatian died. Then the man's world crumbled around him. In a matter of weeks he was dead too.

Few of the dogs that came to me for treatment had done much travelling and for a very good reason. If they went abroad they had to face six months in quarantine when they came back and neither they nor their masters cared much for that.

But Spot, the Comte de Bellissen-Durban's dog, was widely travelled. He was—and happily still is—as much at home in Sierra Leone or the Congo as in Paris or London.

Spot was born in Sierra Leone and there is no mistaking him when you see him. He is a big white cross-bred terrier with two brown spots and brown ears.

The Comte—who is English, despite his ringing French title—worked in Sierra Leone for ten years. For the last eight of them he and Spot were inseparable. The Comte's job took him all over Sierra Leone and he and Spot would travel about three thousand miles a month, the dog lording it in the back of the car. Sometimes friends of his owner's would get in the back with him but he made it quite clear that this was a gross and unwarranted intrusion.

In 1956 the Comte returned to England for three years and Spot followed by a later plane and endured his first six months of quarantine. Then the Comte went to the Congo and again Spot flew out to join him. By this time the Comte had married, and though Spot wasn't enthusiastic about this turn of events he was polite enough to his new mistress while remaining strictly a one-man dog.

These were the years just after independence and the Congo was in turmoil, but Spot liked it there. The climate suited him. Still, there were no complaints when the Bellissen-Durbans packed up again and returned to Europe. This time they lived in Paris for two years and Spot liked it there too.

Then they made yet another move—this time to London, which Spot didn't care for at all. It meant a second six months in quarantine.

Still, that's over now and Spot is enjoying a peaceful old

age. He is more than eighteen and, after one severe heart attack, he is looking his great age. He sleeps a great deal, has grown rather greedy and for the past two years has been stone deaf. The Bellissen-Durbans did think at one time of getting him a canine hearing aid—they make them in America and they work quite well—but decided against it.

His has been a long full life, though I don't suppose the old dog can remember much of it now. He will have long forgotten, if indeed he ever knew, the innumerable puppies he sired up and down Sierra Leone in his young days. He will have forgotten the hit-and-run driver who almost killed him in Freetown, the spitting cobra that blinded him for twelve days, even the boxer who almost killed him in the Congo—though he still bears the scar of that attack.

But such things are commonplace experiences of all old African hands. They happen every day and all the time. Old colonial dogs like Spot, snoozing away their well-earned retirement, have better things to think about. Like what there will be for dinner tonight and how the present generation aren't half the dogs their fathers used to be.

I have known many expensive dogs in my time, but never one so costly as Sir Benjamin Hogg.

Sir Benjamin was a big brown dog, half retriever and half airedale, who wouldn't have won any prizes at Crufts, but he was a dog with a very big personality.

In 1947 an American girl came to England to marry Mr. Edward Hogg. It was her first visit and she didn't like it much. It was wet and cold, the natives were unfriendly and she had half a mind to get the next boat back to the States.

However she had an appointment to see a house in Sussex, so she looked it over and was given tea by the owner. This didn't help much as she hated tea. Then in walked Ben.

She fell for the dog completely. The owner said that the dog went with the house, and from that moment the house was sold.

"The truth is," says Mrs. Hogg, "that my husband bought the house just so that I could have Ben." A *very* expensive dog.

After that Ben went everywhere with her, took her into the village daily, introduced her round. She was a stranger, so the villagers didn't talk much to her, but they all without fail said "Good morning, Ben" as they passed.

The Hoggs came to hate leaving Ben behind to go anywhere—particularly the States, where they would be away for eight or ten weeks.

Once in Chicago they were at a large dinner party at the Yacht Club when, after a few drinks, the hosts told everyone about Ben.

One of the guests insisted that all the bones from their steaks should be sent to Ben by air. The guest's wife was extremely bitter when she learned the cost of this. "I've spent years helping my husband through school," she told the Hoggs, "and this is how he spends our money . . ."

It turned out to be a most elaborate operation. Someone called a United Airlines hostess who agreed to take the bones to New York and connect with a B.O.A.C. hostess who would carry on to England. Everything went wrong with the connections and the bones were delivered three weeks later by a postman holding his nose. They all had to be buried.

Ben was eighteen when I finally had to put him to sleep. I always thought of him as the archetypal squire, a bit old-fashioned in his views, rather grumpy at times but always very, very English.

The country, he clearly thought, was going to the dogs—but not nearly fast enough for his liking.

NINETEEN

The pedigree show dog lives in a curious world. His is a life of constant grooming, training and discipline, of patient waiting and short exciting moments in the limelight. It is a world in which an extra millimetre of tail or the way he carries his head can make the difference between the championship, glory, and an overjoyed owner on the one hand, and utter failure and a glum ride home on the other.

But cups, rosettes and rounds of applause aren't the only rewards for a champion. That extra millimetre of tail and the way he carries his head can mean a lot of money too.

Immediately a dog or bitch becomes a champion, up goes the stud fees, up goes the price of the puppies.

So with both money and honour at stake it is not surprising that the atmosphere round the show ring gets a bit tense at times.

Dogs are sensitive to atmosphere and they react in very different ways. Some beautiful, highly-bred dogs are intimidated by the excitement and are at their worst when being shown. Others love every minute of it.

Boozer, for instance, was in his element. He had only to see a show-lead and he would stand into his best position, one leg stretched well behind, head erect, back elongated, looking every inch a champion.

If I took other dogs to a show and left him behind, he would whine and sulk and have a miserable day.

Watching Boozer, parading for the judges, bags of swank, completely sure of himself, I'd sympathise with some of the nervous dogs competing with him. Some may have been better than old Boozer, but with their tails drooping and their heads down they certainly didn't look it.

When eventually I stepped into the ring myself as a judge for the first time I sympathised even more. I was in an agony of nerves.

Once as a lad of eighteen, I had been cast in a production of *The Middle Watch* which the Old Boys of my school were putting on. The rehearsals were fine but on the night itself I was driving to the hall when all at once I was overwhelmed by stage fright. I could hardly steer the car. So I stopped, did a three-point turn and drove away as fast as I could. I'd let everyone down and was overcome by guilt for days. Now twenty years later I felt the same panic all over again. I shifted from one foot to another, my mouth was dry, my hands no longer seemed to belong to me. If I could have run, I would.

Then the show started and gradually I became absorbed in the dogs. The absurd self-consciousness went and I started to enjoy myself.

Indeed, as the months went by and I got more and more invitations, I began to enjoy judging enormously.

Though I judged many other breeds, in time I specialised

in the three varieties of dachshunds and it was these I judged at Crufts.

Crufts is the greatest dog show in the world and to be asked to judge there is a great honour. It is beautifully organised and exhibitors, as well as their dogs, are usually on their best behaviour.

At smaller dog shows, though, there could be some remarkable displays of temperament.

I got accustomed to being smiled at very sweetly before the judging started and being cut dead when it was over. I got used to getting warm invitations to drinks and dinner and parties weeks before a show from hopeful dog-owning ladies (all of which, of course, had to be declined), and getting flattering letters with photographs of dogs I would be seeing in the ring a few days later.

And after the show I would overhear—as I was meant to —cutting asides in piercingly projected stage whispers. " Of course," I once heard an unsuccessful competitor hiss, " *he dyes his hair . . .*"

I saw one breeder exhibit a dog with its tail pinned to its back with a kirby grip and refuse to take it out. I saw a breeder of French bulldogs push her finger into the exhaust of her car and smear the soot over the face of her champion to make its black face blacker. I saw dogs with noses tattooed black, white-coated dogs powdered so thickly with chalk that if anyone touched them a little white cloud rose in the air.

I've been asked to judge poodles with coats obviously dyed, and I've known several cases where plastic surgery has been used to correct ears and tails.

At one show I smelled burning and, turning, saw an exhibitor singeing the coat of his wire-haired dachshund with a lighted taper.

None of these dodges are much help to a dog in a show ring. Indeed they only put judges off.

The dog shows held every St. Patrick's Day in Dublin were always the most hectic, calling for a strong head and large capacity for whisky. Irish hospitality is irresistible and if poor English dachshund judges didn't have a hangover the day of the show they certainly had one the morning after.

My favourite, though, was always the Everyman's Dog Show which raises money for the Guide Dogs for the Blind.

Any dog can be entered, from the most aristocratic thoroughbred to the most harum-scarum of Heinz 57 Varieties, and everyone entered just for the fun of the thing.

We enjoyed ourselves enormously *and* raised a great deal of money for Guide Dogs. And in all the years I judged there—always on the last Saturday in July—I can't remember the day being anything but dry and sunny.

Bitches on heat should not be entered for dog shows, but sometimes they are and the effect on the general decorum of the dogs all over the hall can be disastrous.

After one show I was sitting in front of a television camera explaining to viewers the winning point of each dog put before me, when a bitch in this condition completely wrecked the programme.

She had been all right in the ring. But perhaps the lights or the heat or the general excitement brought her on, because we were suddenly and alarmingly joined by an ardent prospective bridegroom who started to make love to her in full view of a fair proportion of the population. The programme came to a sudden ignominious end. But we had made television history of a kind. . . .

Boozer conducted his love life a little more discreetly, but no monarch was ever more determined to leave a sufficiency of heirs behind him.

One of his daughters, Sari, who had been mated so successfully with Lady Headfort's Max, came to my kennels every time she was in season. The idea was that she would be out of harm's way.

We reckoned without her father. It was not fatherly love that persuaded Boozer to perform such Herculean feats to overcome all obstacles to reach his child one night. I was awakened by unmistakable sounds, and jumping out of bed I have never moved faster. But too late, too late. Boozer had tunnelled under the wire netting around her kennel and they were together . . .

Deeply embarrassed I had to phone the owner and tell her what happened. In due course five puppies were born, beautiful little dachshunds all the image of Boozer. They grew up strong and healthy with no obvious signs of too-close inbreeding. Indeed one won a third at Crufts.

As for Sari, her career as both nurse and mother came to a macabre end.

I had delivered a litter of three enchanting griffon puppies, worth perhaps £60 each. Their mother wouldn't look at them. Sari had plenty of milk so I called her in.

For ten days she fed them and mothered them and they were making splendid progress. The owner was delighted.

Then, on the eleventh day, we found Sari alone in her bed. There was no sign at all of the griffon pups. We searched for them until the grim truth slowly dawned on us. Sari had eaten them.

The telephone call I then had to make to the pups' proud owner was as difficult a task as I have ever undertaken.

It is hard to explain why bitches sometimes do this fearful thing. All I can say is that, very rarely, they do, eating their own litters to the last pup and clearly not understanding why their owners are horrified and either punish them or, worse, withdraw their affection.

Bitches with a new litter are always unpredictable. Often they will turn against one particular pup, sometimes the strongest and most attractive looking of them all, pushing it away and refusing to feed it. Meanwhile they will be perfect mothers to the wretched outcast's brothers and sisters. There is very little an owner can do about the odd pup out. It usually dies.

Sari was forgiven of course and still visits me, an old lady of fourteen, and she brings her son, Boozer the Second with her. He is a mature gentleman of twelve.

Boozer lived until he was seventeen—a good age for a dog. In his later years he became a terrible old roué and was mating bitches almost to the end. He sired, in his time, more than two hundred puppies.

And here is a remarkable thing. As he grew older he seemed to know instinctively when I was preparing to do a Caesarean operation and would take up his position in a bed under the operating table and wait for each puppy to be delivered. He would lick them clean and nurse and fuss over them until the mother regained consciousness. I have never known another dog do this.

I had to put him to sleep in the end. He had lost his sight and was suffering badly from the ailments of great age and this was the least I could do for such a dear old friend. Again he left a gap in our lives that was hard to fill even with other dogs all round us.

That is the trouble with animals. Their life span is so much shorter than ours that, unless you keep an elephant, a parrot or a giant tortoise, you usually outlive one dearly loved pet after another. It isn't a thing you ever get used to. Indeed I think it gets worse as you get older. You become less emotionally resilient. Your grief takes longer to heal.

I think Wanda missed Boozer almost as much as I did, but she was never low spirited for long.

She loved to come with us to the beach and would sit, blissfully content, piling up stones and loving being the centre of attention.

One day I had left her sitting happily on the balcony of a flat owned by Hal Higgs, my strong right hand for many years. I returned to find Wanda at the top of a lamp-post in the street, screaming at poor Hal who, exasperated and out of breath, was trying to get her down. I drove by and called to her. Immediately she leaped into the car, flung her arms round my neck and welcomed me as if I'd been to China, not just round the corner.

She took a hot-water bottle to bed every night and covered herself completely with a blanket. This, however, was unsatisfactory. It meant she couldn't see what was going on. So she bit two peep holes in the blanket and we would see her eyes watching us, until she dropped off to sleep.

She became increasingly fond of a wee drop to drink and doted on brandy. Indeed she would have become a real old soak if we hadn't kept the stuff locked up.

One night she had a severe heart attack. I at once gave her a teaspoonful of brandy. She took the spoon, put it in her mouth and drank the brandy with murmurs of enjoyment. Then, the spoon still in her mouth, she too died.

There were fifty dogs in the kennels, with twenty-five cats in the cattery. I was surrounded by members of my family, friends and colleagues. But that night I felt lost and utterly alone.

TWENTY

A passion for animals is not, of course, just an English trait. It is something you find wherever you travel.

English vets aren't allowed to practise in many foreign countries, but no one can stop them treating sick animals they meet on their travels and whenever I went on holiday I always took some pills and instruments with me in case they were needed. They always were.

Once, indeed, they got me out of a very embarrassing situation. I was on holiday with some friends in St. Tropez, now a famous international playground but then a quiet fishing village of great charm. It had been a disappointing holiday with the Mistral blowing up and keeping us all indoors, and we were about to return home without a hint of suntan.

Then, on the last day, the Mistral blew itself out and the sun blazed down. We had spent the last of our then meagre allowance but couldn't bear to leave, so we just stayed on. Living there was cheap in those days, but a *few* francs were needed and we hadn't any at all. So I got out some medicines and set up shop in the Hôtel de Paris.

There was no other vet for miles around and the word sped round the village and surrounding countryside. Le Veterinaire Anglais was in attendance.

So the local artists and hoteliers, the restaurateurs and shopkeepers, the fishermen and the farmers streamed to the bar of the hotel with their dogs and cats and goats and cows and horses. The little bar had never seen such customers before.

The sun blazed down, the heat was terrific and there was the beach which I loved but I was far too busy to enjoy any of it. The week passed slowly and the reckoning came. We had our lodgings to pay, but first I had to be paid myself. Well, my grateful clients rolled in, beaming all over their faces, and pressed on me gift after gift. Paintings, pieces of sculpture, antique objets d'art, odd bits of furniture—but no money. Not a franc. Not a cent. I was aghast.

I took the only course possible, set out all the gifts in the Bar Bleu and offered them for sale. Prices were low, trade was brisk, our bills were paid and we could be on our way home again.

On my first visit to Paris after the war a Madame Gold-schmidt-Halot appealed to me for help. All her animals but one had been killed by the Nazis who occupied her apartment, and this, a poodle called Laurette, was the apple of her eye. But it was in an appalling state—covered in sores and bald patches.

I did what had to be done, gave strict instructions about future treatment, and left with some misgivings.

Within a year Laurette was made Champion of France and very soon afterwards International Champion, the highest honour a dog can win. Each time the judges commented on the denseness of her glorious coat.

In Corsica, too, my instruments were needed. On my first night of a holiday there I was wakened by the heart-rending lowing of a cow in pain. I couldn't bear it and next morning I tracked the poor beast down. She was in agony. Her leg and foot were septic and the intense heat and the flies both added to her misery.

The farmer was delighted when I offered to treat his cow every day for nothing, and by the end of my holiday she was almost fully recovered. Cows are nice, friendly animals when you get to know them and this one was most affectionate and grateful and always pleased to see me. So I was all the more horrified when I heard what her future was to be. After all my work she was to be killed and eaten the day after I sailed. . . .

My travels in Europe brought me in touch with some remarkable women—women with names that sound like a fanfare of trumpets.

In Marbella there was the elegant Princess Max de Hohenlohe-Langenburg, mother of Prince Alfonso, and the woman who made the use of unpadded horses in bullrings illegal. She and her son had two hunting dogs and a poodle and one of the hunting dogs had had an unlikely accident. He had chased a bird up a tree, had got wedged in the branches and had dislocated his shoulder. This was easy enough to put right and I heard later that from that time on he left climbing trees to experts. Like cats and small boys.

Then there was the Contesse de Munn whose little Yorkshire terrier had tried to pick up some processionary caterpillars in the Retiro Gardens in Madrid. This is a curious species of caterpillar. They stick together head to tail and look like a long worm. Their bite can be fatal and Moustique just got to me in Marbella in time.

The Contessa Miscatelli asked me to treat her dogs on the island she owned off Porto Ercoli in Tuscany. I expected two or three dogs—half a dozen at the most. But after a long bumpy drive across the causeway I was greeted by an ear-splitting din. The little island was alive with tiny griffons and the arrival of a stranger had set them off in full cry.

They were everywhere, all over the house, running wild on the beaches and in the woods, and I gave up counting them. They are such nippy little creatures that I felt I may well have been counting each of them ten times.

Then there was the Marchesa di Bourbon del Monte who adored pekes. I helped choose a group for her at Crufts and these became the foundation of a wonderful kennel. The Marchesa's pekes are celebrated today. They have swept the board in show rings all over Europe.

Once when I was in Paris for treatment myself she rang me with a most urgent summons. Her pekes were seriously ill, she said. Would I *please* come to Tuscany at once?

I'd no time to get to the bank, but rushed to the airport, caught the next plane to Rome and arrived without a lira. A car met me at the airport and off we went.

I shall never forget that drive, the trees outlined against a sky bright with a huge moon, the sea gleaming silver, the owls filling the night with their eerie music. Then I was being swept into the magnificent villa, welcomed with all the warmth and effusiveness of emotional Italians and whisked out again to the kennels.

The pekes were very ill indeed and needed urgent attention. I started then and there at two in the morning and worked on, almost without respite, for two days.

While I was going flat out in the kennels an archeological dig was going on in the grounds and on the morning after I arrived they started to uncover the most beautiful things. A fantastic bracelet of coloured stones. A beautifully proportioned early Tuscan bowl. Each extraordinary object was shown to me with pride and delight as they came to light. I looked and marvelled and returned to the pekes.

By the time I was through I was light-headed with tiredness. But the pekes were responding and at last I knew for certain that they were out of danger. The sweet relief and deep quiet happiness such rare moments bring are greater treasures than any that were being unearthed outside among the orange trees.

It was in Italy too that I came to know the fabulous Contessa Marina Luling Buschetti Volpi, owner of the famous Villa di Maser, one of the most magnificent houses in the world.

The Contessa is a dazzling woman who wears exquisite rings with pendants of precious stones on the tips of all her fingers. She has more than twenty dogs—pekes, dachshunds, chihuahuas and Irish wolfhounds and at times she would send one of them to me by chauffeur-driven limousine right across Europe for treatment.

And as time went on I found myself writing letters of advice to animal owners all over the world. At one time I had patients in Mexico, the Argentine, Australia, and almost every country in Europe simultaneously.

I even had some patients in Hong Kong—a family of chow-chows owned by a Mr. Chow. I could hardly just nip over to Hong Kong and back, so I never did meet Mr. Chow's chow-chows face to face.

Nor did I ever meet any of the cairns and beagles in

Ontario that I treated by post for twenty years. Their owner —who I never met either—would write to me sometimes every week and would send me cables, describing symptoms, asking what she should do about this and about that. I knew the case history of every one of her many dogs so intimately that I sometimes thought that if I met one of them in the street I would have recognised it at once.

The animal-loving Englishwoman abroad does seem rather a figure of fun seen from this distance. There she goes with her cheerful, well-scrubbed face through the tropics in her tweeds and sensible shoes, berating the natives for ill-treating their camels and getting back to her chintzy verandah in time for tea.

The truth is not like this at all. Englishwomen do crop up in the most distant places and they do, certainly, do their best to stop the locals being cruel to animals. They would have done the same if they had stayed at home. When you meet them they turn out to be amusing intelligent women who fit well into the life of their new countries and who rarely make themselves conspicuous.

Naomi Jacob was rather an exception—but she was an exceptional woman in every way. Short, burly, Eton-cropped and kindness itself, she bulldozed her way through life, never afraid of making a scene or wading in with her gold-knobbed walking stick at the ready.

She campaigned ceaselessly against circuses and performing animals and I was once at the Hippodrome in Brighton when a dog act started on the stage. Immediately a furious figure rose in the stalls and a loud deep voice filled the theatre with protest. "Get those dogs off the stage," she bellowed. And the dogs left the stage. Naomi Jacob usually did get her own way.

She lived for many years on the shores of Lake Garda in Italy and I went there many times to see her dogs.

The local Italians knew her as Signora Micky and were in great awe of her. She went on at them about keeping birds in cages, about overworking mules and donkeys, about tying up their dogs, and the priest there told me that he had seen her attacking a tough in the street with her stick and sending him home with a very sore head. She had seen him kicking a donkey.

I liked and admired her enormously and have fond memories too of her adored pekes, Cup, Saucer and Count Baldo.

When Saucer died Miss Jacob wrote to say that Count Baldo had gone into a black collar that day. " And I," she added, " will wear a black tie for three months."

Then there is Joan Campbell, a good-looking Englishwoman who has settled in Marbella, in the south of Spain. She always has dogs round her and recently started an animal refuge there to cope with any cat or other animal without a home. She gets on with it quietly, but all Marbella knows that if there's an unwanted dog or cat around, Miss Campbell will help.

In Jamaica I met another of these generous, open-hearted women. This was Mrs. Lettice MacNeal. Mrs. MacNeal is short, stout and rich and lives in a beautiful house overlooking the Caribbean.

She loves cats and takes in any stray that needs a home. And what a home they get! Last time I saw her Mrs. MacNeal had forty cats and I hear she now has seventy-two—and they live a luxurious life with rooms in the big house set aside just for them.

There are such women in the most remote, uncomfortable, unexpected places, women whose work for animals is known only to the people of the village or town they live in.

They get little praise, less thanks and no money at all for their efforts. Indeed it usually costs them far more than they can afford.

But they are the salt of the earth, these self-effacing, unknown women—as the animals they befriend soon discover.

TWENTY-ONE

I loved travelling, but my life's work was at Dene's Close and it was always wonderful to get back there, to be greeted by Jackie at the lich gate, by my marvellous staff and by the dogs and cats filling the kennels and cattery.

Looking back on it now I find it hard to account for all the success I had with animals. I can't explain why they immediately quietened under my hands, why they came so happily to my surgery and why after painful illnesses they would eagerly come back to see me.

Nor can I explain now—nor indeed could I explain then—the diagnoses I sometimes made and the treatments I prescribed. There were sometimes cases far outside my training and experience, but somehow I felt instinctively what was wrong and what had to be done.

I don't find this an easy thing to write or speak of. But I had the overwhelming sense of a help that was outside myself, and which grew with the years.

It is hard, too, to describe the peace and tranquillity of Dene's Close. There was rarely enough room for all the cats and dogs that needed to stay there and we all worked long hours and sometimes got very little sleep, but no one minded about that. Those were, for me, the happiest years of my life.

I was surrounded by people who were only too keen to take work off my shoulders—Hal Higgs who did all the accounts, Susan Squire who ran the kennels with meticulous efficiency, Mr. Winton, a train driver who spent all his spare time doing the garden. . . .

One of my patients, a peke called Honey, fell for him completely. She had broken her back and was in plaster and a bit sorry for herself, but the gardener had only to appear for her to cheer up at once.

Eventually she would eat only if he fed her and the dear man came in specially three times a day to do this. Then, when we wanted her to begin walking again, it was once more the gardener who persuaded her to try. And with great success. Honey had been very badly injured, but she recovered completely. She still comes to see me every summer.

During one visit to Rome a young American asked if I would train him as a veterinary dietician. I agreed and he became a great asset to us. His name was Robert Carrier. He has since made a name for himself as an expert on food of a very different kind.

It was a wrench to leave Dene's Close even for a short time, but as my practice grew I had to be away more and more.

I would drive away at the crack of dawn, Diana, my assistant-cum-secretary, by my side, a typewriter on her lap and a stack of correspondence in the glove compartment, on the shelf above the dashboard and on the rear seats. I would dictate and she would type and somehow all the most urgent queries got replied to as we drove through the countryside.

Sometimes we'd go more than two hundred miles to see sick dogs and get home again late at night to find the waiting room crowded.

I never had fixed surgery hours which wasn't very businesslike, but I always liked people to feel I was there if I was needed. I did try to persuade them to ring up first, if only to make sure I wasn't going to be treating kennels in Devon or Yorkshire or Westmorland that day, but a lot of people would turn up on spec and some of these would wait patiently for hours if I was away.

But usually things had quietened down by ten or eleven. The last client would have left, the dogs and the cats would be bedded down for the night, and I would at last have some time for operations.

Midnight would often find me working away at the operating table. Then to bed and up again early next morning.

It was a marvellous life.

Vets are usually warmly welcomed to kennels and farms, but I remember one occasion when I met a stone wall of hostility.

The Canine Insurance had asked me to visit a farm with one of their representatives to see a greyhound. He was a very successful winner and had recently been insured for £2,000. Then almost at once, he had developed paralysis of the hind legs. The farmer who owned him, backed by the local vet, wanted to put him to sleep—and collect the money.

There had been a heavy snowfall during the night and it was bitterly cold. Diana and I put blankets and lots of newspapers—which dogs find even warmer than blankets—in the back of the car and made the long trip to the farm. Just before we arrived I stopped the car and filled three hot-water bottles at a house by the roadside.

The farmer and the insurance man were waiting for me, the farmer very angry. No, I couldn't see the dog, he said. What business was it of mine?

It was, of course, as representatives of the Insurance Company, very much our business and he had to show us where the dog was in the end. He was in a loose box and it was freezing in there. He was in a bad way, unable to move his hind legs at all and he had no protection from the cold.

Diana and I quietly lifted him up and carried him to the car. The insurance man and the farmer were still arguing in the yard and didn't see us. We put the greyhound on the back seat, tucked hot-water bottles around him and covered him with newspapers and blankets and just drove away. I wouldn't have changed places with the insurance man at that moment for anything—but we had to get the dog away. He would have died if he had been left in that loose box.

It took some weeks to get the dog right, but by the time he left the Denes he was completely well again. The farmer got his dog back, the insurance company saved their £2,000 and I was paid my expenses for the journey. My real payment was seeing the greyhound, lithe and strong again, belting full pitch round the paddock at Dene's Close. He was a magnificent creature.

As we were so near the sea a steady stream of gulls and cormorants found their way to my surgery. They would usually be covered with oil from ships and be utterly helpless. These were always urgent cases because these wild seabirds rarely can adapt, even to a slight degree, to any kind of captivity. I would clean off the oil immediately, feed them raw fish—they were usually starving—and would then rush them back to the sea to release them.

Once a swan came in with a broken wing. I set it in plaster and bedded him down in an outhouse. He wasn't very happy, but the wing mended and in a couple of weeks the plaster was off and the swan was back on the pond again, a bit ruffled but able to fend for himself again.

Quite a few bushbabies came in too. They are lovely to look at but tricky to handle. Like all nocturnal creatures, they don't really make very rewarding pets—unless, of course, you are a nocturnal creature yourself.

But most of my patients continued to be dogs—dogs of all kinds, shapes and sizes.

Lord Haig brought me his golden retriever down from Scotland, a beautiful animal called Carissima, and Hermione Baddeley teetered in on the highest of high heels

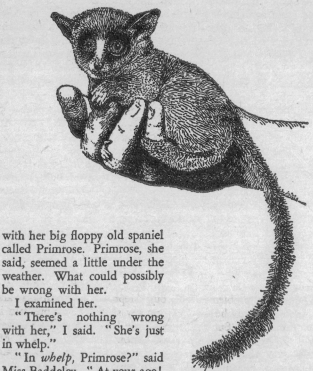

with her big floppy old spaniel called Primrose. Primrose, she said, seemed a little under the weather. What could possibly be wrong with her.

I examined her.

"There's nothing wrong with her," I said. "She's just in whelp."

"In *whelp*, Primrose?" said Miss Baddeley. "At your age! You naughty old thing. . . ."

General Tollemache brought me his devoted springer, Bill, a fine sportsman who still enjoys the shooting season as much as his master, and Alan Melville brought his dachshund, Lily Marlene.

Dora Bryan came with her dear old poodle Sam, who developed cataracts and went blind. It was just old age and nothing could be done to give him his sight back. When at last he died Dora got herself a miniature schnauzer called Fred and she often brings him to see me. Dora signs my visitor's book; Fred leaves his signature on my carpets. "Oooh that Fred," says Dora. "He's done it again!"

Ronald Searle brought his dachshund and stayed to sketch the other owners. One breeder asked me to remove her dogs' vocal cords to stop them barking which I wouldn't and Anton Walbrook brought his pug and asked if I could pos-

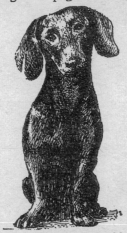

sibly cure it of snoring, which I couldn't. I quite saw Walbrook's problem. The pug slept in his bedroom and snored so loudly he couldn't get any sleep. So he put him in the next room. But the snores came loudly through the wall and still kept him awake. Alas, I know just what it's like. My own pug also snores like a trooper. If you own a pug, snoring is something you have to learn to live with.

As I look back on those years in Dene's Close, it is the peace of the place I most remember, but occasional excitements do stand out.

Late one night, for instance, two of the kennel maids saw the shadow of a man nipping in and out of the trees. They called me and I saw him too. We had a real live burglar on our hands. I called the police and they were with us in minutes complete with tracking dogs.

Alas, among the fifty or so dogs in the kennels that night was one bitch on heat.

In the face of this overpowering new attraction the police dogs forgot all about their mission. They found the bitch all right. Our burglar they never found.

One of the policemen looking across the big heavily wooded garden, very quiet and still in the moonlight, turned to me with some sound police-type advice.

"You know what you need on a big place like this?" he said. "What you need is a dog. . . ."

I vividly remember, too, one chow that came to me late in 1959. He arrived looking bizarre in a pair of flannelette pyjamas. I took them off to find the poor dog almost completely bald.

He had a few hairs on the rims of his ears and a few more on the tip of his tail and that was all.

"I made him the suit because he looked so self-conscious," said his owner. "He must get cold too. . . ."

The baldness was caused by an advanced acid condition and I was most reluctant to take the case on. The condition had gone so far that I suspected it was beyond cure. Several other vets had already come to this conclusion and it looked as if they had been right.

But, against my better judgment, I began treatment. I gave strict instructions about how the dog should be fed and what treatment should be followed, the chow was put back into his pyjamas again and was whisked away in a Bentley.

I heard nothing for four weeks. Then the owner rang in great excitement. She had followed my instructions to the letter, she said, and that morning six new hairs had appeared.

I wasn't too elated myself. Six hairs don't make a chow's coat. But next time the chow came in Susan Squire and I were thrilled to see a down appearing right across his back. And every time he returned his coat was looking better.

It took about a year of treatment in all, but at the end of that time his coat was once again magnificent.

Indeed, a few months ago the owner rang me, very

apologetically. She realised, she said, that this was a strange request, but could I please do something to thin the coat out a bit? It was too dense for comfort.

I remember this chow particularly because he marked a milestone in my life.

A chow had been my first patient all those years ago. And another chow was now proving to be almost my last.

TWENTY-TWO

There is one aspect of my life I haven't talked of much. But now, reluctantly, I must.

Ever since that childhood attack of polio ill health had plagued me. Each stage of my career was interrupted by spells in hospital, some short, some not so short. I was passed from doctor to doctor, specialist to specialist, and all the time I knew in the back of my mind, that one day, one awful, distant day, I might have to give up my practice. But that was some time far in the future. It didn't bear thinking about.

The periodic illnesses became steadily more severe, but I survived one crisis after another. I was out of patience with illness. I had no time for it. I had too much work waiting for me in the real world outside. And after each spell in hospital I couldn't wait to get back to the animals and forget myself. If I helped the animals, they certainly helped me.

Early in 1958 I began to lose the use of my right leg. This was a great nuisance, but I had it in callipers and was able to get around. I was always a very fast driver and loved powerful cars, but now I couldn't manage them. I kept on getting smaller and smaller cars until even a tiny convertible was too much for my legs. Then I got myself a disabled driver's car with the brakes, the gears and the clutch all operated by hand. I found I had to take another test to drive this car and was very insulted. I had, after all, been driving cars all my life. But I took the disabled driver's test, passed it and carried on.

But the strength in my arms was going too. I just couldn't

145

cope with a car any more. So I got someone to drive me.

One day a specialist came to see me at Dene's Close. He admired the place immensely, as, indeed did everyone who saw it. "It's beautiful here," he said. "It's like being in the heart of the country. But you'll have to leave. It's the worst place for you. The trees take all the oxygen and you won't be able to walk up the hill from the lich gate much longer. . . ."

He said it in that matter-of-fact way specialists have. I was shattered. I thought it was a bad dream and told no one what he had said. I tried to forget it, but it wasn't an easy thing to forget.

I toyed with the idea of selling the practice altogether. Quite a few vets were keen to buy and one came down with a very good offer. I almost took it. Then he started asking questions.

"How much does she pay?" he said, nodding to an elderly woman whose dog I was treating for canker. "Not much," I said. "She can't afford it."

"That's one I'll get rid of," he said. "And what about him? How much does he pay?" He pointed to a client of long standing, a retired man with only his old-age pension, who brought in his mongrel and his Norwich terrier whenever they weren't well. "He doesn't pay anything," I said.

"That's another one who'll have to go," he said.

It seemed all wrong. I remembered it was *people* and their animals I was selling, not just a house, a garden and a lot of equipment. How can you sell people?

"I'm sorry," I said. "I've changed my mind. The practice is not for sale. . . ."

Then I became really ill again. I was in bed for four months. Diana and Susan brought dogs and cats up to me and I examined them from my bed, diagnosed their ailments, gave instructions about treatment.

Jackie, my beloved golden retriever, had passed away and for the first time in my life I had no dog of my own. So Mary Kessell sent down Annabelle, her golden retriever, to keep me company.

For Annabelle it was like coming home again. She was one

of Cleo's litter of eleven and had actually been born in the bedroom I was now lying in.

All her life Annabelle had loved coming back to see us all at Dene's Close. She always stayed with me, for instance, on the night of November 5th—and so did several other golden retrievers. They are placid, sweet-natured dogs but they are exceptionally upset by sudden noises. There were bangs around Dene's Close too on Guy Fawkes' Night but somehow the dogs felt safe there and could observe the progress of a battery of squibs and Moon Rockets without alarm.

Now she ran into my bedroom, smiling, swinging her tail and giving me her paw, and for the next few weeks she spent hours by my side and cheered me up while I lay there thinking about my future.

Obviously I couldn't carry on just as before. But perhaps I could go on in a limited way. So I had plans drawn up for the conversion of the house into flats and got planning permission from the council to go ahead. The idea was that I should live on the ground floor and run a greatly reduced practice from there. I would need a new surgery and waiting room, so I had these built in the garden—very modern and beautifully equipped.

The surgery and waiting room were finished in September. In October I went into hospital. My doctor said I needed a thorough check-up but it wouldn't take long. Ten days at the outside. I'd be in and out before I knew it.

So I made appointments to see clients in ten days' time, gave instructions about treatments for patients in the kennels, packed an overnight bag and cheerfully left.

I never saw Dene's Close again.

The ten days became a fortnight, then a month, then two months, then three. And something happened to me in those three months that made this an illness unlike any I had ever had before. I had had a power with animals. I have already written of it. Now I felt it being switched off just like that, click, as you would turn off a light. The power had gone. It has never returned.

TWENTY-THREE

Much against my will, I've become quite an expert on hospitals. I've been a patient in so many.

I can now distinguish between a plate of hospital rice pudding and hospital tapioca at ten paces and can usually tell their tea from their coffee just by the taste—though this takes much practice. I can tell the chink of the injection trolley from the clink of the food trolley. I know what it means when the corridors fall suddenly, breathlessly silent, I could write the definitive text-book on hospital bedmaking techniques, and lying in hospital bed after hospital bed I have worked out the exact composition of the universal hospital smell—a smell which, as a matter of fact, I rather like. Indeed, this is the only thing about a hospital that I do like.

I've been in big hospitals and small, old hospitals and new, good hospitals and bad. I was in a French hospital where the food deserved at least one star in the Michelin Guide and in an American hospital where my room was on the twenty-fourth floor and had pictures on the walls which were changed every day. This is the only glamorous hospital I know. The nurses would have survived only about five minutes on the staff of an English hospital, but I had to admit that they were exceptionally chic.

The nurses in the hospital I now found myself in weren't particularly chic but they were wonderfully efficient, dedicated and hard-working. The hospital itself, on the other hand, was the worst I have known.

It was—indeed it still is—a famous chest hospital with an international reputation and marvellous work has been done there. But the brilliant specialists on the staff have to work in a complex of buildings that should have been bulldozed years and years ago. Things may have improved there in the past five years, but nothing less than complete rebuilding would really do the trick. The buildings are ancient, ramshackle, makeshift, badly planned and hopelessly outdated.

The sanitary arrangements when I was there were disgraceful and to the windward side of my room was a highly active factory chimney, the contents of which saturated the air. Every morning I awoke to find my bed covered with a fine layer of best quality soot. The only way to prevent this was to keep the windows closed. But with the windows closed I couldn't breathe at all. So, for the whole time I was there I breathed in sooty air day and night.

In my ten weeks there I grew progressively worse. When, just before Christmas, I was finally released, my career as a vet was over. For the rest of my life I was to be in a wheelchair and it was clear that I could never work again.

The day my dear friends Dorothy Pearson and Hal Higgs came to collect me I was so full of drugs I didn't know who they were or who I was. The doctors told them I had three months to live.

Their immediate problem was where to take me.

They couldn't take me to Dene's Close with its trees, its long climb to the house, its corridors and its stairs. They couldn't take me to the charming Regency cottage that had been prepared for me in Brighton. We had fitted in an expensive new spiral staircase which made it impossible. So we went to an hotel.

It wasn't a very merry Christmas.

The Christmas cards that were sent for me that year almost tore me apart. One went to each of my two thousand regular clients. They announced the closing of Dene's Close and the end of my career.

They explained that I was too ill to carry on. And I added that this was only a temporary measure, that after a year, perhaps, I might be able to start again. I prayed with all my heart that this might prove to be true.

My devoted staff split up and dispersed. The dogs in the kennels and the cats in the cattery went back to their owners. The furniture in the house went into store and Susan, the last of the rearguard, locked up and went off to London to run Dene's, the shop which sells the natural foods and remedies for animals that I had devised and used for so long.

Now the lovely old house stood empty again and in the

gardens only the birds and the small wild creatures of the countryside stayed behind.

All that remained for me to do now was to get as well as, under the circumstances, I could. I was told that sunshine would help. And that the world's greatest authority on chest diseases practised in New York. So Dorothy, Hal and I set off for Jamaica, calling at New York on the way.

I was wheeled aboard the *Queen Mary* and spent most of the voyage in my cabin, being looked after by the ship's doctor and nurse. New York was cold and crisp and sunny with snow thick on the ground, the air wonderfully clear and invigorating and very good for me.

We had booked into an hotel that overlooked Central Park, thinking it would be easier to breathe there than in an hotel in one of the downtown canyons of that hectic city. At once we realised our mistake. The hotel had steps from the street to heavy, plate-glass swing doors and then more steps to the lobby. A man in a wheelchair can't manage either steps or swing doors and it was our rare misfortune to find that the doorman, a surly young chap, wouldn't help at all. He not only declined to give a hand with the chair but refused to even hold the door open. It was a bad beginning.

Still, I saw the world's greatest authority and he raised my spirits to dizzy heights.

He examined me and said there was nothing wrong with me that he couldn't put right. He would have me walking upstairs again in six months, he said. But first, he said, go off and have your holiday in the sun.

We were elated. In a moment New York was transformed into the most wonderful place on earth. We loved everything about it and everyone in it. We even loved our unfriendly hotel doorman.

We packed again and, elated and thankful, took a slow boat to Jamaica.

We had taken a heavenly house on the Caribbean called Blue Horizon. The weather was superb, the people delightful and soon I found myself actually treating a few animals again. Dogs in Jamaica are prone to digital cysts which trouble them a great deal and I dealt with several of these. Then there were Mrs. MacNeal's cats to be looked at and a pathetic little dachshund which had been badly cut about with a machete. I made many friends and they urged me to stay on and run an animal refuge there.

But I was only operating at half throttle. It wasn't the same somehow. The extra thing I had had only a few months earlier, the spiritual help, had gone.

What's more my mind for once, wasn't on my work. I was counting the days to get back to New York, to hospital, to the great man I had built up such faith in. I believed with all my heart that this was going to be the final cure.

We had planned to return to New York as we had come, by sea, but all the boats from Jamaica were delayed by a shipping strike. So, while Dorothy and Hal stayed on board with the luggage, I got off at Miami to complete the journey by air.

It was the first time I'd ever been on my own in a wheel-chair and I found the prospect extremely exciting. It was, however, to prove a far more involved journey than any of us expected.

Friends had arranged for me to be met at Miami docks and shown round the town. My guide turned out to be a pleasant, courteous young man, who drove me round all morning, wined and dined me at the airport restaurant and then put me in the V.I.P.s' lounge to await the plane. I then insisted that he leave me there. He'd already given up almost the whole of his day. Nothing, I said, could possibly go wrong now. So he said goodbye and I was left alone. Time passed and before long I began to find it impossible to catch my breath. The air-conditioning in the room was absolutely over-powering.

I was eventually found slumped in my wheelchair in a state of collapse, my oxygen cylinder slung over my shoulder.

I was revived, only to hear that my plane had been cancelled. There were, it seemed, terrible electric storms ahead. So everyone rallied round to help me. I was whisked away to an hotel and someone was detailed to be with me all the time. Five hours later the storms subsided, I was collected from the hotel, rushed back to the airport and wheeled across the tarmac where, to my astonishment, a bevy of photographers started clicking away.

I couldn't imagine what was happening. Then I looked round and there were about fourteen other people in wheelchairs behind me. Apparently there had been a wheelchair conference in Miami that week and I had got myself in the middle of one of the delegations.

At last I was on the right plane, going, however, to the wrong city. The electric storms started up again and the plane had to put down at Philadelphia. Again people rallied round and I was wheeled aboard another plane which got me to New York hours late, exhausted but buoyed up by the knowledge that the great man was awaiting me.

I stayed in an hotel that night and next day was moved into a bed in the great man's hospital overlooking the Hudson River. The hospital was hugely expensive. So was the great man. His fees, as you might imagine, were astronomical. Anyone who ever criticises the National Health Service should try being ill in America.

The treatment was much the same as I'd had in London and Paris. It made me feel progressively worse. Again I was meant to be there for just a few days. This crept up to a month and I was still there and still no better.

At last the great man said he was sorry. There was, after all, nothing he could do.

I was numb with disappointment. After all my hopes I could scarcely believe it. But I had to believe it. I paid his bills and got myself out of there as quickly as I could.

Now we couldn't wait to get home. We got berths on the first ship out of New York harbour and made the worst journey of my life. The ship creaked and tossed and lurched its slow way to Southampton while I lay in my berth and faced a future that seemed empty and without hope.

I was at my lowest ebb.

TWENTY-FOUR

As England drew nearer my spirits rose again. Dorothy and Hal insisted that the three of us should make a new life together and were full of plans for the future. I sometimes wonder if they knew what they were taking on. But gradually I caught their enthusiasm and once again rediscovered my old appetite for life.

All the doctors agreed that what I must have at all costs was sea air, so back we went to Hove to look for a place where all three of us could live. We each already had a house of our own and very pleasant houses they were, but none was any use to a man permanently in a wheelchair.

Almost at once we found that the penthouse of a big block of flats right on the seafront was vacant. We looked round it and could hardly believe our luck. It was ideal. No stairs, no narrow doors, no corridors with awkward turns.

Three sets of furniture came out of store. Some had to be discarded, the rest polished up and given, like me, a new lease of life.

At last we were settled in and could begin the awful business of selling Dene's Close.

It was, for some reason, a bad time for selling. It always is when it's your turn to sell as perhaps you've noticed. Dorothy's house sold quickly enough but Hal's Regency cottage, which had cost a lot, hung fire and then went at a big loss. And Dene's Close didn't go at all.

So we put it up for auction.

Going to the auction rooms that day was like going to a funeral. I hated it. But I went all the same.

Not many were there, and of those who did attend few were serious bidders. The price rose slowly. "Going, going, gone," said the auctioneer and knocked it down to Dorothy!

I don't know whether I was more horrified or surprised. "I only wanted to push them up a bit," she said, horrified too.

But Dorothy Pearson is a woman of resource. She was the

English Ladies' Golf Champion. She has played bridge for England. International golfers and bridge players are not easily flustered. She had a quiet word with the auctioneer and Dene's Close, the house I loved so much, went at a bargain price to the last bidder but one.

I have never been back. I couldn't ever bear to. I have never met the lady who bought it. But I hope she is happy there and I hope that she has dogs and cats and perhaps a tortoise or two to share it with her.

It is, after all, a house that has grown accustomed to animals. Somehow I don't think it would feel right without them.

Certainly I felt lost without animals around me and as soon as it was possible I bought a stalwart little pug puppy called Puddy. He finds it perfectly natural that I should move on wheels and not on legs and a dear friend he has been to me from the start.

Then I found myself a successor to Pollyo—a fine green parrot called Polly, a talented talker and a great laugher. He can out-laugh anyone in the room. With a dog and a parrot around I began to feel more my old self. And when I got myself a little electric runabout I felt a new man. This was a joyful possession. I could be helped into it and then speed away along the front under my own steam once more. It was wonderful.

Alas, these runabouts have handles which you have to turn, and after perhaps half an hour my arm would pack up and I'd be stuck far from home. Someone would have to turn out and rescue me. So in the end the runabout was relegated to the garage. I haven't be able to use it for a couple of years now.

But even without my own steam I still get about. Indeed since my life in wheelchairs began I have been almost all round the world. I have been four times to New York. I've been to South America, to many parts of the Caribbean, to South Africa, and to a good many countries in Europe. I'm not allowed to fly now—air travel plays havoc with my dodgy lungs—but I can still go places by boat and so the world is still there at my doorstep.

I don't *like* being in a wheelchair, of course, but I've come to terms with it. Indeed, it's only when I meet another man in a wheelchair that I remember I'm in one myself.

Wherever he goes a man in a wheelchair meets with astonishing kindness from complete strangers. I have, all the same, had my share of embarrassing moments.

When I was in Las Palmas, the year before last, for instance, I was left for perhaps fifteen minutes sitting in my wheelchair outside a church. The sun was dazzling and I was wearing very dark glasses and was carrying a small leather sachel containing passports, travellers' cheques and so on. A coach drew up and I watched, lazily, while about thirty or forty cheerful tourists got out, chattering and laughing. Suddenly, to my astonishment, I found coins being pressed into my hands. For a moment I couldn't think what was happening—and then it dawned on me. These good souls thought I was begging. I was horrified and couldn't wait for my friends to come back and get me out of there. As soon as they appeared they wheeled me rapidly to a bar where I recovered my holiday spirits over a good stiff drink.

Every now and then, when the weather is bad or the mist comes in from the sea or for no good reason I can see, I am suddenly laid low again and am rushed to this hospital or that clinic.

One such visit was a great deal shorter than was intended. I had been rushed off in an ambulance to the emergency ward of one of the local hospitals. This was a frightening place. The poor fellow in the bed on my right died during the day and the one on my left was obviously dying too. I knew I'd die if I stayed there.

All day I lay making my plans for escape and, as the visiting hour approached, I prayed that Dorothy wouldn't be wearing a bright red coat. She arrived, all smiles and sandwiches and fruit, in a nice unnoticeable camel-hair. "Put your coat on me," I said urgently. "Now help me into the chair and PUSH." She didn't hesitate for a moment. Right down the full length of the ward we went, not looking to left or right, through the double doors, along the corridor, out the front door and into the car.

Fifteen minutes later we were being welcomed home

again by Puddy and Polly. I've never been more relieved to see them.

But it is always wonderful to get home again wherever one has been, to return to the ordinary small pleasures of everyday life.

I get out as much as I can. I go to the local theatre on occasions and sometimes to the cinema. I'm often asked to parties of various kinds and I go as often as I can though this can be difficult. You'd be surprised how choosy a wheelchair

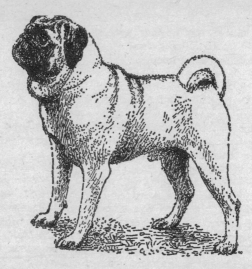

can be. It won't go down area steps to basement flats. It won't go up stairs of any sort. It won't go through doors that are too narrow and it won't even consider revolving doors, come what may. It likes lifts but rejects escalators on sight Wheelchairs are touchy things.

Attending parties in a wheelchair can be great fun though I must admit there are occasional disadvantages.

Perfectly sensible people bend over, their faces close to yours, and talk in very simple terms as to a baby in a pram. No one has ever actually called me diddums yet, nor have they patted me on the head, but they've come pretty near.

Other people tend to lean comfortably on the back of the chair which feels, if you are in the chair, as though the fellow's whole weight was on your shoulders. Then again you can be cornered by the dullest man in the room and be utterly unable to escape. You are the perfect captive audience.

Still, there are advantages too. However crowded the room is, for instance, you, at least, always have a place to sit.

We wheelchairers have our own unwritten code of behaviour. We always, for instance, nod to each other as we pass. And if we meet we talk of many things but never our illnesses. We're a bit sick of that subject.

And so must you be too. So I'll leave it at that.

TWENTY-FIVE

The flat I live in is big and it is comfortable. It has a fine winter garden, four roof terraces and wonderful views whichever way you face.

In one direction you can look across the rooftops to the South Downs. In the other you see the lovely Regency squares and terraces of Hove and Brighton and the cliffs of Newhaven beyond. On a fine day you can see Beachy Head. On the dullest day you can see Brighton's twin piers. Under the windows are the lawns on which the bucks of the Prince Regent's court once strutted, and of course there's always the sea, never the same two hours' running.

For hours at a time I watch the people—the youngsters jumping from the breakwaters into the sea, the families picnicking on the grass, the grandparents walking slowly along the front. Then there are the dogs of Brighton. Every day they come to rollick along the seafront.

I know most of them by sight and many of them by name, for quite a lot of them were once my patients. Or their fathers or their fathers' fathers were. It makes me feel like Mr. Chips. Sometimes a dachshund will run past and I'll know at once it is one of Boozer's many grandchildren. " Ah, yes," I'll think. " That's Boozer's head all right, and that's his back and wouldn't the old boy be proud to see you now. . . ."

People who come to see me always admire the views. "It must be lovely living here," they say. "You never need go out. . . ."

It *is* lovely living here. They're right about that. But you do need to go out all the same. You need, above all, to feel you are being of some use to someone. I'm not, by nature, a spectator. I like to be doing things. I like to be down there among the people and the dogs. Above all I long to be looking after animals again.

Thankfully I have a great many friends who come to see me, bringing news of the great world outside. They often bring their dogs and sometimes their cats too. I had a snake in to tea the other day and a very well-mannered fellow he was.

Sometimes people bring sick dogs in too, but as I'm not in practice now there's nothing I can do. I just have to send them away. This is very upsetting.

Letters come from all over the world and sometimes the telephone will ring and it will be a call from Switzerland or Spain or Paris—old clients wanting help with their animals.

I would dearly love to be able to refer them to another vet carrying on where I left off. Alas, I don't think there is one.

There is still the firm of veterinary herbalists in London with Susan in charge and they carry on my work to a certain extent. But I leave no disciples behind me, no keen young vets who believe, as I believe, that sick animals respond best to natural cures.

Over the years many young students wanted to work with me, to learn my methods. I was always reluctant to teach them. There was too much to do. I hadn't the time. . . .

I bitterly regret this. I know I failed them. But it is too late now.

I'm never allowed to feel I'm forgotten. Last Christmas, for instance, I got more than six hundred cards, many from people whose pets I treated years and years ago and have never seen since. And people are always writing to say they are calling their new puppy Buster, after me. There must now be hundreds of little Busters running round England. All, let me say at once, dogs.

And I have a new interest in my retirement—I've started to keep tropical fish. I have more than a hundred of them now, dazzling, lovely little creatures living a fascinating life of their own. Then there is Bert, an amiable rock tortoise I brought back from South Africa last year.

I was there to miss the English winter which always lays me low and a steward on the ship produced Bert one day to keep me company. He's quite a lively little chap is Bert. He lives on the terrace but pops in from time to time. He has a particular affection for the bathroom for some reason. I'm very fond of him.

It is a small family of animals. Too small. I'd like a few more dogs, and a cat or two. I'd like some monkeys and a fruit bat and a little bantam would be agreeable. A porcupine would be welcome as well, and a donkey to graze in the winter garden and what about a handsome python and those lion cubs I looked after all those years ago on Wimbledon Common.

I would like them all around me now as I sit here writing. But I mustn't ask too much. I have, after all, a dog, a parrot, a tortoise and about a hundred fish. I have devoted friends. I have an operatic doctor who sings arias in a rich baritone as he treats me. And from the window I can see at this minute two golden retrievers in the sea and a labrador, a peke and a cross-bred terrier romping on the lawns.

One way and another I'm a very lucky man.

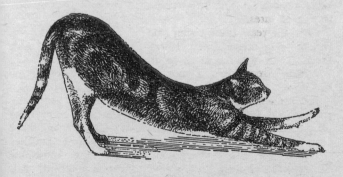

Fontana Books

Fontana is best known as one of the leading paperback publishers of popular fiction and non-fiction. It also includes an outstanding, and expanding section of books on history, natural history, religion and social sciences.

Most of the fiction authors need no introduction. They include Agatha Christie, Hammond Innes, Alistair MacLean, Catherine Gaskin, Victoria Holt and Lucy Walker. Desmond Bagley and Maureen Peters are among the relative newcomers.

The non-fiction list features a superb collection of animal books by such favourites as Gerald Durrell and Joy Adamson.

All Fontana books are available at your bookshop or newsagent; or can be ordered direct. Just fill in the form below and list the titles you want.

_____

FONTANA BOOKS, Cash Sales Department, P.O. Box 4, Godalming, Surrey, GU7, 1JY. Please send purchase price plus 7p postage per book by cheque, postal or money order. No currency.

NAME (Block letters)
_____

ADDRESS
_____

_____

_____

While every effort is made to keep prices low, it is sometimes necessary to increase prices at short notice. Fontana Books reserve the right to show new retail prices on covers which may differ from those previously advertised in the text or elsewhere.